Can Food-Based Strategies Help Reduce Vitamin A and Iron Deficiencies?

Can Food-Based Strategies Help Reduce Vitamin A and Iron Deficiencies?

A Review of Recent Evidence

Marie T. Ruel

International Food Policy Research Institute
Washington, D.C.
December 2001

ISBN 0-89629-504-4
Library of Congress Cataloging-in-Publication Data available.

International Food Policy Research Institute
2033 K Street, NW, Washington, DC 20006-1002, USA
Telephone: +1-202-862-5600; Fax: +1-202-467-4439
www.ifpri.org

Contents

Tables

Box

Foreword

Micronutrient malnutrition is still a problem of unacceptable proportions in developing countries. Iron and vitamin A deficiencies are the most widespread nutrition deficiencies in the world today, affecting perhaps as many as 3.5 billion people. Because they disproportionately affect children and women during their reproductive years, these deficiencies hinder the development of human potential and nations' social and economic development.

It is now well recognized that no single strategy—or "magic bullet"—exists to eliminate micronutrient deficiencies globally. Supplementation, fortification, agricultural interventions, and education to improve dietary quality are all necessary but insufficient approaches. Coordination between sectors is crucial. Multidisciplinary teams must join together to design and implement global strategies to attack the problem in a sustainable way.

Investments in reducing micronutrient malnutrition have traditionally focused disproportionately on supplementation and fortification programs and policies to the detriment of food-based approaches, which focus on increasing the amount of micronutrients consumed in the diet and on making a larger share of these nutrients bioavailable (readily absorbed by the human body). Food-based approaches are complex and require collaboration between a variety of sectors, including agriculture, nutrition, education, and economics. They are long-term strategies because they usually involve significant behavior changes on the part of the recipients, and thus they may need to be implemented and evaluated over periods of 5 to 10 years. Because donors are usually driven by the need to demonstrate impact quickly, supplementation and fortification approaches have often been given priority over food-based interventions in research funding. And their expense and complexity frequently has discouraged researchers and donors from carrying out the necessary in-depth evaluations of food-based approaches. As a result, a dearth of information exists on their efficacy and effectiveness. Without conclusive evidence on how well these approaches work, donors continue to hesitate to invest in large-scale programs.

Although they are indeed long-term strategies, food-based approaches are essential to the fight against micronutrient deficiencies. Of all the strategies, they probably require the highest level of initial investment, but they are also the only ones that hold a promise of sustainability. The evidence presented in this Food Policy Review highlights the key role of education in ensuring the success of food-based approaches. Changing people's behavior in terms of the foods they grow and eat and how they prepare and process them requires a significant amount of effort. It is, however, the only way to enable people to take ultimate responsibility for the quality of their diet.

Per Pinstrup-Andersen
Director General

Acknowledgments

The author thanks Carol Levin for her contribution to earlier drafts of this document; Anna Winoto for her assistance in reviewing and compiling the literature; and Jay Willis for his support with word processing and editing. Support for this review was provided by MOST, the micronutrient program of the U.S. Agency for International Development, and the International Food Policy Research Institute.

Summary

Throughout the developing world, poor people subsist on diets consisting of staple foods such as rice or maize and little else. The lack of diversity in the foods they eat often leads to micronutrient deficiencies. Lack of iron, which causes anemia, is the most common deficiency in the world. Iron deficiency is harmful at all ages, but it especially affects women of reproductive age and children. Vitamin A deficiency impairs growth, development, vision, and immune systems, and in severe cases can lead to blindness and death. Almost one-third of children in developing countries are affected to some degree by vitamin A deficiency and many more are iron deficient.

Micronutrient deficiencies can be addressed by distributing vitamin and mineral supplements, by fortifying foods, or through food-based strategies, which attempt to modify people's diets. Food-based strategies can increase the amount of vitamin A and iron available for body functions by (1) increasing the production and availability of foods high in these nutrients, (2) increasing consumption of these foods through nutrition education programs to change eating behavior, (3) making vitamin A and iron more easily absorbed by the body (more bioavailable), and (4) by breeding new varieties of plants that contain larger amounts and more bioavailable micronutrients.

This report reviews a number of recently published studies of food-based interventions to reduce vitamin A and iron deficiencies in developing countries. It summarizes the current state of knowledge and identifies the lessons learned and the research gaps that remain.

Vitamin A is available from animal sources in the form of retinol and from dark green, leafy vegetables and yellow and orange noncitrus fruits and vegetables in the form of provitamin A carotenoids. Vitamin A from plant sources is less easily absorbed and utilized by the human body—it is less bioavailable—than the vitamin A coming from animal products. In developing countries, most of the vitamin A consumed comes from plant sources and thus is in a less bioavailable form. Moreover, vitamin A from plant sources is usually found in large amounts in only a few fruits and vegetables, many of which are highly seasonal. This means that low-income populations may suffer from both chronic mild-to-moderate vitamin A deficiency and severe seasonal deficiencies.

Iron can also be obtained from both animal and plant sources. Iron from plants (nonheme iron) is less bioavailable than iron from flesh foods (heme iron) such as meat, fish, and poultry. Heme iron is highly bioavailable (15–35 percent is absorbed), whereas iron from plant sources (nonheme) is absorbed much less easily (only 2–20 percent is absorbed). The main reason for the lower absorption of iron from plant sources is that nonheme iron is affected by compounds present in plant foods that inhibit iron absorption. The most potent inhibitor of nonheme iron absorption is phytic acid, which is present in large quantities in most cereals and legumes—often the main staple foods in populations with scarce resources.

This review shows that increasing the availability of foods rich in vitamin A and iron by encouraging households to tend home gardens and to raise small animals and fish is a popular approach. Increasingly, the food-based strategies combine a variety of intervention components. A key to success appears to be the inclusion of a strong nutrition education and behavior change intervention. For example, strategies to promote increased production of micronutrient-rich foods are more effective when combined with a nutrition education intervention, which ensures that increased household food supply and income translates into improved dietary quality.

Proper processing and storage of plant products, in order to retain vitamins and minerals and to extend the time when fruits and vegetables are available—through drying, for example—are other ways to boost consumption of essential nutrients year-round. Cooking in iron pots can increase iron intake. Eating certain combinations of foods together—such as citrus fruits rich in vitamin C and iron-containing cereals and legumes—helps increase the absorption of iron from plant staples. Conversely, not ingesting substances that are known to inhibit absorption with meals, such as coffee and tea, may increase the bioavailability of iron from plant sources. All of these strategies are well documented and are even part of the cultural background of some populations from developing countries, but large-scale, community trials documenting their effectiveness are surprisingly few. Plant breeding approaches, which hold great promise for contributing to the fight against micronutrient deficiency, are still at an early stage of development, and their efficacy and effectiveness have to be demonstrated.

Although the technologies and strategies examined in this review potentially address many concerns about the intake and bioavailability of vitamin A and iron among impoverished populations, enormous information gaps still exist concerning the efficacy and the effectiveness of most of the strategies reviewed, even approaches as popular as home gardening promotion. Significant progress has been achieved in the past 10 years in the design and implementation of food-based approaches, particularly the new generation of projects that integrate production, nutrition education, and behavioral change strategies. Yet, little has been done to assess the impact of these combined strategies on the diets and nutritional status of at-risk populations. In the end, the same question posed in reviews published decades ago remains: what can food-based interventions to control vitamin A and iron deficiency really achieve? Food-based approaches are an essential part of the long-term global strategy to alleviate micronutrient deficiencies, but their real potential has not been explored adequately.

Chapter 1

Introduction

Balanced diets are not accessible to a large proportion of the world's population, particularly those who are poor and live in developing countries. Many people subsist on diets based on cereal staples and little else. Such diets lack diversity (and sometimes quantity), which may result in micronutrient deficiencies. Among the nutritional deficiencies, lack of sufficient amounts of vitamin A and iron have the greatest impact on public health. Almost one-third of children in developing countries are affected to some degree by vitamin A deficiency, which may impair their growth, development, vision, and the functioning of their immune systems: in extreme cases lack of vitamin A leads to blindness and death (UN ACC/SCN 1997; WHO 1995; Sommer and West 1996).

Iron deficiency, which may cause anemia, is well recognized as the most common dietary deficiency in the world (including developed countries). It mostly affects children and women of reproductive age (Gillespie 1998). It is estimated that more than half of all pregnant women in the world and at least one-third of preschool-age children suffer from anemia, and many more are iron deficient to some degree (UN ACC/SCN 1997). Iron deficiency is harmful at all ages. In young children it may impair physical growth, cognitive development, and immunity; in school-age children, it may affect school performance; in adulthood, it can cause fatigue and reduced work capacity. In pregnant women, severe anemia may cause fetal growth retardation or low birth weight, and it is responsible for a large share of maternal deaths (Gillespie 1998). Because iron and vitamin A deficiencies disproportionately affect children and women during their reproductive years, they hinder both the development of individual human potential and national social and economic development.

An existing body of knowledge and experience can be drawn on to address vitamin A and iron deficiencies effectively, using either short- or long-term interventions or a combination of both. The most popular approaches are distribution of supplements, food fortification, nutrition education, and the so-called "food-based strategies."

Food-based strategies—also referred to as dietary modifications—encompass a wide variety of interventions that aim to (1) increase the production and availability of and access to foods high in vitamin A and iron; (2) increase the consumption of foods rich in these micronutrients; or (3) increase the bioavailability of the vitamin A and iron in the diet; that is, the amount of vitamin A and iron that can be absorbed and utilized by the body. Examples of interventions to achieve these goals include the following:

- *Strategies to increase the* production *of micronutrient-rich foods.* These strategies include agricultural programs and policies to increase commercial production of fruits and vegetables and to promote home gardens, small livestock production, and aquaculture (fish ponds).

- *Strategies to increase the* intake *of micronutrient-rich foods.* These approaches refer to nutrition education, communication, social marketing, and behavioral change programs designed to guide consumer food choices and to increase the demand for micronutrient-rich foods. They also include preservation and conservation techniques such as solar drying or production of leaf concentrates to extend the availability of micronutrient-rich seasonal fruits and vegetables throughout the year.[1] Cooking in iron pots is also a strategy to possibly increase iron intake.

- *Strategies to increase the* bioavailability *of micronutrients.* These include promotion of home-processing techniques such as fermentation or germination to increase the bioavailability of micronutrients, and combinations of foods that, when eaten together, increase the bioavailabiltiy of certain micronutrients. (This latter strategy is also called food-to-food fortification.)[2]

---

[1]Breastfeeding promotion programs and education interventions to improve complementary feeding practices are also important strategies to increase the intake of micronutrient-rich foods by specific target groups. Although they are a key component of the global strategy to control micronutrient deficiencies, they are not reviewed in the present document.

[2]Food-to-food fortification also refers to strategies to incorporate micronutrient-dense foods into traditional preparation of dishes that are poor in micronutrients. In this case, food-to-food fortification implies increasing micronutrient intake, rather than bioavailability. Recent experience with the use of such approaches to increase vitamin A intake is reviewed in Underwood (2000) and is not discussed in the present document.

- *Plant breeding strategies.* Plant breeding technologies are also included in food-based strategies because they may (1) increase the concentration of certain trace minerals and vitamins; (2) increase the bioavailability of micronutrients by reducing the concentration of substances that inhibit the absorption of nutrients; or (3) increase the concentration of substances that promote absorption.

In practice, most food-based strategies use some combination of these four groups of interventions. For example, nutrition education and communication strategies can complement production interventions to ensure that increases in food supply or the income from marketed surplus, will in fact, translate into increased nutrient intakes by the targeted groups.

Food-based strategies are often described as a sustainable approach because the process empowers individuals and households to take ultimate responsibility for the quality of their diet by growing their own nutrient-rich foods and making informed consumption choices. These strategies are said to be "the ideal long-term goal toward which society strives—provision of assurance of access to a nutritionally adequate diet achieved through diversity of food availability, wise consumer selection, proper preparation, and adequate feeding" (Howson et al. 1998, 21). Food-based strategies are also appealing because they can address multiple nutrients simultaneously, including energy, proteins, and various micronutrients, without the risk of antagonistic nutrient interactions or overload.

This review summarizes current knowledge and experience with food-based approaches, discusses some of the lessons learned and the gaps in knowledge that remain, and identifies research priorities. It is structured as follows: Chapter 2 looks at the relevant issues related to intake and bioavailability of vitamin A and iron in developing countries; Chapter 3 reviews strategies to increase production or intake of vitamin A and iron; Chapter 4 focuses on strategies to increase bioavailability, with a special emphasis on iron; and Chapter 5 reviews plant breeding approaches. The final chapter summarizes lessons learned and priorities for future research.

Chapter 2

Vitamin A and Iron Intake and Bioavailability in Developing Countries

To successfully develop food-based strategies to combat vitamin A and iron deficiencies, researchers require a thorough knowledge of the sources of these nutrients and how the human body uses them. What foods contain vitamin A and iron? Are nutrients from some foods more readily absorbed and used than others? Can the bioavailability of foods be increased?

Vitamin A

Vitamin A is available from animal sources in the form of retinol or retinol esters, and from plant sources, particularly fruits and vegetables, in the form of provitamin A carotenoids. There are approximately 50 known active provitamin A carotenoids, of which beta (b)-carotene makes the largest contribution to vitamin A activity in plant foods (McLaren and Frigg 1997). Alpha (a)-carotene and b-cryptoxanthin (mainly from fruits) also contribute substantial amounts to some diets. Until recently, it was assumed that the activity of b-carotene was one-sixth that of retinol and the activity of other carotenoids was one-twelfth that of retinol (FAO/WHO 1988). Recent findings suggest that the bioavailability of carotenoids in fruits and vegetables may be much lower than previously estimated (dePee et al. 1995; dePee and West 1996; dePee et al. 1998b; Jalal et al. 1998). The bioconversion ratios in spinach, for example, have recently been estimated to fall between 33:1 and 73:1, as opposed to 12:1 (IVACG 1999). The Reference Dietary Intakes (RDIs) recently released by the Institute of Medicine (2001) recommend using the following conversion factors: 1 retinol activity equivalent (RAE) = 1 microgram (m g) of retinol, 12 m g of b-carotene, 24 m g of a-carotene, and 24 m g of b-cryptoxanthin.

Based on a review of recent literature, Underwood (2000) also proposes a hierarchy of carotenoid bioavailability based on a relative ranking of foods, rather than on specific conversion factors. According to this classification leafy green and yellow or orange vegetables are at the lower end of bioavailability, whereas yellow or green fruit and red palm oil are at the higher end. In developing countries, most of the vitamin A is ingested from fruits and vegetables. Estimates suggest that more than 80 percent of dietary intakes of vitamin A in Africa and Southeast Asia, for example, are from provitamin A carotenoids (WHO 1995).

Because of the current uncertainty regarding the bioavailability of provitamin A carotenoids, the potential of plant sources to significantly improve or even maintain vitamin A status in deficient populations is being questioned by nutrition practitioners. One of the purposes of the present review is to shed light on this question by reviewing the experience to date with the use of food-based approaches to control vitamin A deficiency. Here both interventions promoting plant sources of vitamin A (fruits and vegetables) and those focusing on animal products are reviewed.

Iron

Iron is present in both heme form (in flesh foods such as meat, fish, and poultry) and in nonheme form (in dairy products, eggs, and plant foods such as beans, cereals, nuts, fruits, and vegetables). Heme iron is highly bioavailable (15 to 35 percent is absorbed), whereas nonheme iron is much less bioavailable, with absorption rates ranging from 2 to 20 percent (Allen and Ahluwalia 1997). The factors that affect the amount of iron absorbed from a meal include the individual's iron status and requirements, the sources and content of iron in the meal, and the other constituents of the meal. Absorption of both heme and nonheme iron is affected by the individual's characteristics, but nonheme iron is particularly sensitive to the presence of inhibitors of iron absorption such as phytic acid, tannins, and selected dietary fibers (Hallberg 1981). Ingestion of ascorbic acid and even small amounts of meat and fish, on the other hand, actively promotes absorption of nonheme iron (Fairweather-Tait 1995).

Staple crops provide a large proportion of the total daily intake of energy and micronutrients among poor populations who have limited access to animal foods (Allen et al. 1992; Ferguson et al. 1989). The main sources of iron in these populations—staple cereals and starchy roots, tubers, and legumes—are in the nonheme iron form and have low bioavailability (Gibson 1994). Estimates indicate that cereals contribute up to 50 percent of iron intake in households from lower socioeconomic groups in developing countries (Bouis 1996). The main problem with diets based on staple foods from plants is that they usually contain large amounts of phytic acid, which is the most potent inhibitor of nonheme iron absorption (Gibson 1994; Allen et al. 1992). Therefore, strategies to reduce the concentration of phytic acid in the diet should receive high priority. In looking at food-based approaches, it is crucial to increase the bioavailability of nonheme iron and to increase the total amount of iron absorbed from plant-based diets. Such strategies, as well as strategies that aim to increase the intake of animal products, are reviewed in subsequent chapters.

Chapter 3

Strategies to Increase Production and Intake of Micronutrient-Rich Foods

This chapter summarizes experiences with food-based strategies designed to increase either the production or intake (or both) of micronutrient-rich foods, with an emphasis on vitamin A and iron. It reviews recent interventions that promote increased household production of micronutrient-rich foods through home gardening, small animal husbandry, and aquaculture, as well as interventions that focus mainly on education and other efforts to promote changes in dietary patterns. Strategies to retain more vitamin A during processing and storage and to increase iron intake by cooking food in iron pots are also reviewed.

Production and Education Interventions

On the one hand, vulnerable households may not include nutritious foods in their diet because they are not readily available at the community or household level. Therefore, strategies to increase production and availability of such foods could be effective. On the other hand, household supply, availability, and access may be sufficient, but lack of knowledge and awareness of the importance of consuming nutritious foods may lead to poor diets. That situation calls for strategies that promote the intake of micronutrient-rich foods through education. Because both of these assumptions are clearly simplistic, in recent years many micronutrient interventions have adopted a more holistic approach, combining production and education activities.

Vitamin A Strategies

Home gardening has been the most popular food-based strategy for the control of vitamin A deficiency, and a number of studies evaluating its success have been published over the years. The first of these evaluations was a series of reviews supported by the Vitamin A Field Support Project (VITAL) of the International Life Science Institute (Peduzzi 1990; Soleri, Cleveland, and Wood 1991; Soleri, Cleveland, and Frankenberger 1991), which reviewed more than 40 publications and looked at the impact of home gardens on consumption, nutritional status, and in some cases income. More recently, the United Nations Administrative Committee on Coordination-Subcommittee on Nutrition (ACC/SCN) reviewed 13 dietary modification programs to control vitamin A deficiency, covering work published between 1989 and 1993 (Gillespie and Mason 1994). This volume updates this work and reviews 14 new projects carried out in developing countries and published between 1995 and 1999.[3] Table 1 summarizes the design, intervention, and evaluation characteristics of each study as well as the key findings. Evidence of the impact of these interventions on three main outcomes—production and income; knowledge, attitude, and practices and intake of targeted foods and nutrients; and nutritional status indicators—is presented in subsequent sections.

Impact on Production and Income. The literature indicates that most home gardens are implemented to increase household production of fruits and vegetables as a way of supplementing the grain-based diets of rural agricultural households (HKI/AVRDC 1993; CARE/Nepal 1995; Greiner and Mitra 1995; Solon et al. 1979; English et al. 1997; English and Badcock 1998; Kidala, Greiner, and Gebre-Medhin 2000; Chakravarty 2000). Thus, the main objective of home gardening initiatives is to improve both household food supply and dietary quality. There are also reports of projects whose purpose is to increase households' total food supply mainly during lean seasons (Immink, Sanjur, and Colon 1981), while others aim to increase the availability of micronutrient-rich vegetables and fruits throughout the year (Marsh 1998). Few reports on home garden projects mention the objective of increasing household income through the sale of products or of increasing women's control over income, even in cases where the intervention is mainly targeted to women.

Only a few studies looked at the effects of home gardening promotion programs on household food production. A commonly used indicator to measure the impact on production is the number of households who have adopted garden cultivation

---

[3]The review is restricted to studies conducted in developing countries. For examples of similar studies carried out among vulnerable groups in developed countries, see Kuhnlein and Burgess 1997 and Kuhnlein 1992.

as a result of the intervention. In Nepal and Bangladesh, for example, the proportion of households producing vegetables and (in the case of Bangladesh) fruits increased as a result of home gardening and farming education interventions (CARE/Nepal 1995; Greiner and Mitra 1995). In Tanzania, an agriculture intervention promoting the production of vegetables rich in provitamin A carotenoids increased the percentage of households with home gardens and of households producing such vegetables, compared with a control area (Kidala, Greiner, and Gebre-Medhin 2000). In India, an increase in the percentage of households cultivating dark green, leafy vegetables and other vegetables was documented following a home gardening and nutrition education intervention (Chakravarty 2000).

Few studies have measured actual increases in the quantity of fruits or vegetables produced, although a number of studies have shown an increase in the availability of such foods in households that produced them, compared with nonproducers (English et al. 1997; English and Badcock 1998; IFPRI et al. 1998; Marsh 1998). The projects reviewed by Marsh (1998) in Bangladesh also showed an increase in the year-round availability of vegetables among communities targeted by a home gardening project, compared with control communities.

Only a few studies have looked at the impact on income, farmer's profits, or household market sales. A study by IFPRI and collaborators (1998) in Bangladesh examined the profitability of vegetable or fish production, compared with rice, and linked this to changes in household income. The study showed modest increases in income as a result. Also in Bangladesh, Marsh (1998) documented an increase in household income and in women's control over income as a result of efforts to promote home gardening. An earlier evaluation by Brun, Reynaud, and Chevassus-Agnes (1989) of a project in Senegal also found that home gardens had a positive impact on women's income. In Tanzania, a solar dryer promotion program documented that 8 percent of women in the intervention group used the dryers, but the percentage of women selling dried vegetables did not increase (Mulokozi et al. 2000).

In sum, although relatively few studies have quantified the impact of home gardening projects on household production, income, and women's control over income, those that have seem to indicate a positive trend.

Impact on Knowledge, Attitude, and Practices, and on Intake of Vitamin A-Rich Foods. Efforts to integrate strategies to promote changes in behavior along with home gardening were notably absent in many of the studies conducted in the 1970s and 1980s. Interventions tended to focus mainly on increasing adoption of a particular agricultural strategy and on promoting food production, but the role of nutrition education and communication was largely neglected (Ensing and Sangers 1986; Brun, Reynaud, and Chevassus-Agnes 1989). Not surprisingly, most of those

Table 1. Summary of intervention and evaluation designs of recent studies reviewed

			Intervention		
Country	Reference/ year	Target nutrients	Production	Nutrition education (NED)	Target groups
Vitamin A—Production Intervention with Nutrition Education					
Bangladesh	Greiner and Mitra 1995	Vitamin A	Home gardening Seeds Farming education	NED	Women Children
Bangladesh	Marsh 1998	Vitamin A	Vegetable home garden Agriculture training Seeds	NED	Women Children
Kenya	Hagenimana et al. 1999	Vitamin A	Introduction of new variety of sweet potatoes Training in food processing techniques	NED to increase intake and use of processing techniques	Women's groups Children 0–5 years
Ethiopia	Ayalew, Wolde Gebriel, and Kassa 1999	Vitamin A	Agriculture training Food preparation Seeds	Health education NED	Women Children
Tanzania	Kidala, Greiner, and Gebre-Medhin 2000	Vitamin A	Agriculture, promotion of home production of VA-rich foods Consumption, storage of VA-rich foods	Health education NED	Women Children
Tanzania	Mulokozi et al. 2000	Vitamin A	Solar dryers promotion	Nutrition and health education	Women

(1995–99)

Evaluation		Findings			
Design	Methods	Production	Income	KAP + Dietary intake	Nutritional status
Treatment/ control Before/after	HH survey Clinical assessment 24-hour recall	Increase in % HH growing vegetables and fruits in both treatment/ control	n.a.	Increased knowledge of function of VA	Slight decrease in night blindness
Treatment/ control Before/after	HH survey Vegetable production Size of cultivated plot Income Intake of vegetables	Increase in vegetable production Increase in size of plot cultivated Increase in year-round availability of vegetables	Increase in income Increase in women's control of income	Increase in vegetable consumption per capita Increase in vegetable consumption of children	n.a.
Treatment/ control Before/after	HH survey HKI VA food frequency KAP	n.a.	n.a.	Greater HKI score for frequency of intake of VA-rich foods in children (control group had decreased intake)	n.a.
Participants/ nonparticipants After	HH survey Qualitative research HKI VA food frequency	n.a.	n.a.	Treatment area had better KAP about VA, night blindness; More diversified diet; Higher HKI VA food frequency scores	Treatment area had lower prevalence of night blindness and Bitot's spots
Treatment/ control After	HH survey 7-day frequency recall intake of VA-rich foods Serum retinol Stool analysis (helminths)	Treatment area had hHigher % HH with home gardens; Higher % HH producing VA-rich vegetables	n.a.	Treatment area had better KAP about VA; Higher % HH drying VA-rich foods (solar dryers or shade); Higher 7-day frequency of intake of VA-rich foods	Treatment area had lower serum retinol; Higher helminths; Greater frequency of intake of VA-rich foods (DGLV) associated with greater serum retinol
Treatment/ control Before/after	HH survey (demographics, vegetable availability, food drying prac-	8% of women in intervention group adopted dryers (adopters	No significant increase in income from selling green vegetables	HKI results significantly higher in treatment group; no increase in intake of plant foods,	n.a.

(Continued)

Table 1. —Continued

Country	Reference/ year	Target nutrients	Intervention: Production	Nutrition education (NED)	Target groups
			Business training		Children (VA intake)
India	Chakravarty 2000	Vitamin A	Home gardening	Nutrition and health education	Household (specific age groups not specified)
Niger	Parlato and Gottert 1996	Vitamin A	Promotion of home production	Multimedia education campaign to promote increased intake of VA-rich foods (season-specific): liver, DGLV, squash, mangoes	Women Children
Vitamin A—Production Intervention without Nutrition Education					
Nepal	CARE/Nepal 1995	Vitamin A	Home gardening Irrigation Agriculture extension Seed distribution	n.a.	HH Children 6–60 months

Evaluation		Findings			
Design	Methods	Production	Income	KAP + Dietary intake	Nutritional status
	tices, income-generating activities, expenditures) HKI VA food frequency Child anthropometry (baseline only) Knowledge about solar dryers, VA	appear to have higher socioeconomic status) No significant increase in % HH selling dried vegetables		however; increase was in intake of animal products (result of NED) HKI results higher among adopters compared with non-adopters (within intervention group)	
Before/after	HH survey Weekly consumption of VA-rich foods (method not specified) Ocular signs of vitamin A deficiency	% HH cultivating DGLV increased Production of all types of vegetables increased	40% of HH sold 10–25% of the produce	Increased % of HH felt that cultivation of papaya and DGLV should be increased Increased awareness of importance of DGLV for young children Increased knowledge of symptoms of VA deficiency Weekly intake of DGLV increased at HH level (more than doubled)	Reduction in ocular signs and symptoms of VA deficiency (conjunctival xerosis, Bitot's spots, night blindness)
Before/after (not specified)	Exposure to media intervention Knowledge Intake	n.a.	n.a.	Increase in women who cited VA-rich foods as important for child health Increased intake of DGLV (children) Increased purchase and intake of liver (women and children)	n.a.
Before/after	HH survey	Increase in percent of households producing vegetables	n.a.	Insufficient VA intake by mothers and children both before and after	Deterioration of nutritional status of children during study period (no control)

(Continued)

Table 1. —Continued

Country	Reference/ year	Target nutrients	Intervention: Production	Intervention: Nutrition education (NED)	Intervention: Target groups
Vitamin A—Nutrition Education Intervention without Production Component					
Indonesia	de Pee et al. 1998b	Vitamin A	n.a.	Social marketing campaign, including mass media, face-to-face communication to increase intake of DGLV and eggs	Mothers Children <36 months
Micronutrients—Production Intervention with Nutrition Education					
Viet Nam	English et al. 1997 English and Badcock 1998	Vitamin A Vitamin C Iron Iodine Proteins, calories Fat	Home gardens Fishponds Animals	NED	Mothers Children <6 years
Thailand	Smitasiri and Dhanamitta 1999 Smitasiri et al. 1999	Vitamin A Vitamin C Iron Iodine	Seeds distribution Farmer women training Promotion of gardens, fishponds, chicken raising	NED Social marketing	Pregnant, lactating women Children 2–5 years School girls

Evaluation		Findings			
Design	Methods	Production	Income	KAP + Dietary intake	Nutritional status
Before/after	HH survey 24-hour recall Biochemical analysis	n.a.	n.a.	Increased percent of children and mothers who ate at least 1 egg in past week Increased amount of vegetables prepared per person per day Increased VA intake of children and mothers Increased VA intake from eggs and plants	Serum retinol increased (more egg consumption) Dose-response relationship
Treatment/ control After	HH survey Morbidity recall KAP Anthropometry Food intake	Treatment group had greater production of vegetables, fruits, fish, eggs	n.a.	Treatment group had better KAP; Greater intake of vegetables, fruits, energy, proteins, vitamins A and C, iron in children	Treatment group had lower severity and incidence of ARI; Better growth of children
Treatment/ control Before/after	HH survey 24-hour recall Biochemical assessment (in school girls)	n.a.	n.a.	Increased KAP about VA, iron Increased intake of VA in all target groups No increase in fat intake Increase in iron intake in 2–5 year olds, 10–13 year olds, and lactating women Increased intake of vitamin C in lactating women	Blood samples in school girls: -increased serum retinol -reduction in VA deficiency -increased mean hb (not significant) -reduced anemia prevalence (not significant) -reduction in low serum ferritin

(Continued)

Table 1. —Continued

			Intervention		
Country	**Reference/ year**	**Target nutrients**	**Production**	**Nutrition education (NED)**	**Target groups**
Micronutrients—Production Intervention without Nutrition Education					
Bangladesh	IFPRI et al. 1998	Vitamin A Iron	Vegetable production Fishponds Credit and agricultural training	n.a.	Women Their household and children
Micronutrients—Nutrition Education without Production Component					
Peru	Carrasco Sanez et al. 1999	Vitamin A Vitamin C Iron	n.a.	NED in community kitchen Capacity building	Nonpregnant women of reproductive age

Notes: DGLV = dark, green, leafy vegetables; HKI = Helen Keller International; HH = household; KAP = knowledge,

studies that looked at the impact on food intake or nutritional status failed to demonstrate any significant change in these outcomes (Brun, Reynaud, and Chevassus-Agnes 1989; CARE/Nepal 1995).

By 1994, things had started to change. Gillespie and Mason (1994) in their review noted that more behavior change and communication projects were being implemented, either as the main intervention or in combination with production activities. They highlighted two successful nutrition education and social marketing interventions using mass media that showed a positive change in knowledge, attitude, and practices: one carried out in Indonesia (Pollard 1989) and the other in Thailand (Smitasiri et al. 1993). In Indonesia, positive changes in attitude about consumption of vitamin A-rich foods occurred among targeted mothers who had heard radio spots (42 percent); consumption of dark green, leafy vegetables increased by 10 to 33 percent after two years among the targeted group. Coverage of a vitamin A capsule supplementation program also increased from 35 to 58 percent, as a result of an increase in demand instigated by a social marketing program (Pollard 1989). In Thailand,

Evaluation		Findings			
Design	Methods	Production	Income	KAP + Dietary intake	Nutritional status
Three groups: fishponds, vegetables, control Before/after	HH survey Anthropometry Biochemical analysis	Increased production of vegetables and fish	Slight increase in income from adoption of fish or vegetable technology	No increase in consumption of fish among fishpond group Increase in vegetable intake among vegetable group	No effect on hemoglobin from fishponds or vegetable production
Members/non-members Before/after	Interviews Focus groups Biochemical assessment	n.a.	n.a.	Increased quality of meals (VC, VA) Increased intake of foods rich in iron, VC Increased intake of VC, heme iron, proportion of absorbable iron	Reduction in prevalence of anemia

attitudes, and practices; n.a. = not available; NED = nutrition education; VA = vitamin A; VC = vitamin C.

increased knowledge and awareness about vitamin A in target communities resulted in increased intake of a locally consumed dark green, leafy vegetable called ivy gourd and fat (both of which were promoted by the social marketing campaign) among pregnant and lactating women and preschool-age children (Smitasiri et al. 1993). In 1996, a follow-up to this project was implemented, which again relied heavily on social marketing techniques to promote community-based actions to increase micronutrient intake by vulnerable groups, specifically pregnant and lactating women, schoolgirls, and children two to five years of age (Smitasiri and Dhanamitta 1999; Smitasiri et al. 1999). The evaluation showed that there was a cumulative improvement in knowledge, attitude, and practices with respect to vitamin A and fat consumption among participating communities, whereas no change was observed in the control group. Improvements in knowledge, attitude, and practices were accompanied by an increased intake of vitamin A among preschool-age children and pregnant and lactating women in program areas. Increases in vitamin A intake were also observed among the control group, but they were generally of smaller magnitude.

Another social marketing campaign promoting increased intake of dark green, leafy vegetables and eggs in Indonesia (de Pee et al. 1998a) documented an increase in the percentage of children 12 to 36 months of age who had consumed at least one egg in the previous week. The quantity of dark green, leafy vegetables prepared at home also increased from 93 to 111 grams per person following the intervention, and the total vitamin A intake of both mothers and young children increased. This study did not have a control group, so estimated differences were based on before and after comparisons.

A unique education and behavior change project in Peru to increase the quality of the meals offered in community kitchens (*comedores populares*) of Lima showed a significant increase in the vitamin A, iron, and vitamin C content of the meals provided (Carrasco Sanez et al. 1998). As a result, the intake of foods rich in these micronutrients increased among women using the community kitchen and also the proportion of absorbable iron found in their diet.[4]

Among the home gardening interventions with strong education and behavior change components, several documented an increase in vegetable consumption as a result of the project. One of these was a project undertaken by Helen Keller International and the Asian Vegetable Research and Development Center in Bangladesh, where average weekly vegetable consumption per capita increased among target households, compared with a control group (Marsh 1998). Intrahousehold consumption data also showed that infants and very young children consumed more dark green, leafy vegetables than those in the control group. In Viet Nam, a community nutrition project combining promotion of household production of carotene-rich fruits and vegetables, fish ponds, and animal husbandry with nutrition education showed that participating mothers had a better understanding of vitamin A than mothers from the control community (English et al. 1997; English and Badcock 1998). In addition, children from participating households consumed significantly more fruits and vegetables and had greater intakes of energy, protein, vitamin A, and iron. In India, a nutrition education and home gardening project increased knowledge of the signs of vitamin A deficiency, such as ocular symptoms, as well as awareness of the importance of dark green, leafy vegetables for weaning-age children (Chakravarty 2000). Household intakes of dark green, leafy vegetables more than doubled among participants following the intervention.

In Kenya, new varieties of sweet potatoes rich in beta-carotene were introduced to women's groups (Hagenimana et al. 1999). The control group participated in on-farm trials and received minimal agricultural support for the production of the new varieties of sweet potatoes, whereas the intervention group received nutrition education, lessons on food processing, and technical assistance. The intervention group experienced a statistically significant increase in the frequency of consumption of vitamin A-rich foods, compared with a decrease in the control group.

In Ethiopia, a home gardening and health and nutrition education intervention was built into an existing dairy goat project. The evaluation showed that study participants had greater knowledge about the importance of vitamin A consumption and how to prevent night blindness (Ayalew, Wolde Gebriel, and Kassa 1999). Changes in attitudes and practices were accompanied by increases in the frequency of intake of vitamin A-rich foods. Note, however, that the nonparticipants had lower incomes, and analyses did not control for such potentially confounding factors. Therefore, differences in intake of vitamin A-rich foods should be interpreted with caution.

Two projects carried out in Tanzania, one promoting the use of solar drying to preserve food (Mulokozi et al. 2000) and the other combining horticultural activities and nutrition and health education (Kidala, Greiner, and Gebre-Medhin 2000), documented more frequent intakes of vitamin A-rich foods.[5] Interestingly, the increases in vitamin A intake found in the solar dryer promotion project (Mulokozi et al. 2000) resulted from increased intakes of animal products, rather than from dried vegetables or fruits. This finding indicates that the nutrition education component of the intervention, which promoted increased intake of vitamin A from all sources, was more successful than the solar drying intervention itself in increasing vitamin A intakes.

In Niger, a 10-month multimedia campaign promoted increased consumption (and production for some products) of four vitamin A-rich foods depending on seasonal availability (Parlato and Gottert 1996). These included liver, dark green, leafy vegetables, squash, and mangoes. Intake of liver among participating women and children increased markedly as a result of the intervention, and the overall purchase of vitamin A-rich foods more than tripled.

Overall, the studies reviewed consistently show the success of well-designed promotional activities using nutrition education, social marketing, and mass media campaigns (with or without home gardening) to achieve significant increases in the consumption of micronutrient-rich foods (vitamin A in particular). Compared with the home gardening interventions carried out in the 1980s, which did not include education activities, the new generation of integrated production and education projects have been much more successful in improving knowledge, awareness, attitude, and practices related to vitamin A.

---

[5]The horticultural and education intervention (Kidala, Greiner, and Gebre-Medhin 2000) documented increases in intakes of vitamin A-rich foods, but it did not specify whether the increase was due to greater intakes of the specific foods targeted by the intervention.

Impact on Nutritional Status. Although the question of whether home gardens have a positive impact on vitamin A status has been examined in a number of reviews, including some recent studies, evidence is still scant. In the earlier studies, home gardens were positively associated with a decreased risk of vitamin A deficiency (Cohen et al. 1985) and clinical signs of vitamin A deficiency in eyes were reduced (Solon et al. 1979). A review by Gillespie and Mason (1994) also concluded that food-based approaches could be effective in the control of vitamin A deficiency. In the review of recent work undertaken for this report, only a few of the home garden and nutrition education studies actually measured the impact of such projects on vitamin A status indicators. In Bangladesh, Greiner and Mitra (1995) documented a slight reduction in night blindness associated with an increase in intake of dark green, leafy vegetables in young children. They found that consumption of dark green, leafy vegetables had increased significantly in project communities while decreasing in non-intervention areas. Also in Bangladesh, higher intakes of eggs and dark green, leafy vegetables among children and mothers were associated with greater serum retinol levels (de Pee et al. 1998a). Note that both studies report associations between intake of vitamin A-rich foods and vitamin A status, but they do not systematically evaluate the effects of the interventions.

Compared with baseline levels, decreases in ocular signs of vitamin A deficiency (conjunctival xerosis, Bitot spot, and night blindness) were also documented in India, following a home gardening and nutrition education intervention (Chakravarty 2000).

In Thailand, where serum retinol was measured only among school-age girls, significant increases in retinol were observed among the treatment group, and the prevalence of vitamin A deficiency was reduced (Smitasiri et al. 1999). The social marketing intervention, however, also included a strong school lunch improvement component. Thus, it is not possible to determine which specific aspects of the intervention were associated with the improved vitamin A status.

In Viet Nam, serum retinol levels were not measured, but the prevalence of stunting and the severity and incidence of acute respiratory infections were reduced among children who lived in the area included in the intervention. These improvements were associated with a program that combined the promotion of home production of vegetables, fish, and livestock with nutrition education (English et al. 1997; English and Badcock 1998). In Ethiopia, the prevalence of eye problems such as night blindness and Bitot spot was lower among participants in the home gardening and nutrition education intervention, compared with a control group (Ayalew, Wolde Gebriel, and Kassa 1999).

Evaluation of the home garden and nutrition education intervention in Tanzania showed no difference in serum retinol levels between the treatment and control groups after five years of intervention (Kidala, Greiner, and Gebre-Medhin 2000). The evaluation, however, did not have baseline information. The authors hypothesize that one potential explanation for the lack of positive impact from the intervention may be the high levels of helminth (parasitic worm) infestation among children in the treatment area. Overall, a strong association was found between higher helminth levels and lower serum retinol; when data on children from the treatment and control groups were combined, those with helminths had a mean serum retinol almost half that of children who were not infected. When the comparison of treatment and control groups was restricted to children without helminths, however, differences in serum retinol between the two groups were still statistically nonsignificant. The authors caution that program evaluations should take confounding factors into consideration, and they highlight the importance of measuring and controlling for helminth infestation in evaluations of vitamin A interventions.

Conclusions on Vitamin A Strategies. Consistent with the earlier reviews, this synthesis of more recent literature finds that home gardening and promotional and education interventions clearly have the potential to improve vitamin A nutrition, especially when they are combined. Compared with previous interventions, most recent home production projects include strong education and communication components. Some recent projects have no production component at all, but instead are designed specifically to promote increased intake of micronutrient-rich foods through social marketing and communication activities. Many interventions also rightly emphasize the needs of small children and pregnant and lactating women. It should also be noted that some projects are designed to address multiple micronutrients, not just vitamin A, as in earlier studies.

It is striking, however, to realize that five years after Gillespie and Mason's review, with an addition of more than a dozen new, apparently successful studies, we still do not have sufficient information to understand the real potential of these interventions to control vitamin A deficiency. The new studies have focused on community participation aspects and on the careful selection of appropriate sets of interventions for specific contexts. They also use considerably improved design and implementation strategies. The evaluation protocols and the statistical analyses of findings, however, remain weak and often lack scientific rigor, even in the recent work (see the box for a description of weaknesses in evaluation designs and proposed solutions to improve them). Failure to correct this crucial aspect will continue to slow down progress in understanding the real potential of production and education interventions to control vitamin A deficiency.

Common Evaluation Problems and Solutions for Improving Impact Analysis of Food-Based Interventions

In this review, the main design, evaluation, and analysis flaws encountered fall under three categories: (1) lack of replicate units of intervention and analysis, (2) inappropriate selection of control or comparison groups, and (3) inappropriate control for confounding factors and intermediary outcomes. A brief summary of the implications of these evaluation weaknesses is presented here, followed by suggestions for improving the evaluation of food-based interventions.

Lack of replicate units of intervention

Many food-based interventions are evaluated by comparing a single geographic area that receives the intervention with another area that does not receive it (referred to as the control area). The evaluation compares the situation in the intervention and control area before and after the intervention. The problem with this approach is that changes that occur in either the treatment or control area independent of the specific intervention being evaluated are not considered. This makes it impossible to attribute changes in outcomes to the intervention. Take, for example, a strategy to promote vitamin A intake, which combines increased production of vitamin A-rich foods and an education intervention to increase awareness of the importance of vitamin A for young children. Assume that the assessment of impact is based on differences in the changes in mean serum retinol values between the treatment and the control areas. Findings show that serum retinol values improved more in the control area than in the treatment area. Why? Perhaps changes in weather conditions or other natural trends occurred or other interventions may have been put in place in one study area and not the other during the follow-up period. If, for example, a vitamin A supplementation program was implemented in the control area one year before the follow-up evaluation, interpretation of the findings relating to the difference in serum retinol values between treatment and control areas will be flawed. The absence of replicate units of observation (other geographic areas with and without treatment) makes it impossible to assess the real impact of the food-based intervention independently from the supplementation program.

Recommendation: To avoid this problem, replicates of intervention and control areas should be included, so that fundamental differences between areas can be averaged out, including differences in baseline conditions and later differences arising from unobserved or uncontrollable natural phenomena or development interventions. Care must also be taken to collect detailed baseline and postintervention information on the characteristics of the areas so that "area effects (or community effects)" can be controlled for in the analysis.

Inappropriate selection of a control or comparison group

Many of the studies reviewed include a control group, but little information is provided on how the control group was selected and how comparable it is to the treatment group. Random selection of participants is seldom feasible for large-scale, food-based strategies. Problems arise when detailed information is not collected on communities and households included in a control group to ensure that the two groups are comparable.

Another common approach to the selection of a so-called "control" group is to use a group of nonadopters in interventions where participation is voluntary. This approach is particularly popular for interventions that involve production activities because households cannot be forced to engage in the activities being promoted; thus participation or adoption is self-selected. The problem with this approach is that individuals and households who decide to adopt an intervention or take part in a program may be inherently different from those who do not. It is common, for example, for those who are extremely poor to exclude themselves from production activities or from interventions promoting new crop varieties either because they do not own the land to engage in these activities or they cannot afford the risk associated with adoption of new varieties.

Recommendation: The problems of noncomparable control groups and self-selection seriously affect the validity of the comparisons made between control and treatment groups. Thus, care should be taken to select comparison groups that are as similar as possible in all aspects other than their participation in the program. Since self-selection of adopters and nonadopters may seriously invalidate the findings of the study, care should be taken to gather detailed information on the characteristics of the two groups, so that differences between them can be addressed statistically. Statistical analysis, however, cannot fully control for the problem of self-selection. Therefore, when self-selection is an issue, alternative approaches should be used to select treatment and control groups.

Inappropriate control for confounding factors and intermediary outcomes

The previous points highlight the importance of gathering information on the households and communities being compared to ensure that if differences exist, they can be addressed, at least partially, by controlling for these differences in the analysis. The evaluation studies reviewed generally lack in-depth information on potential confounding factors. Even more important, the studies that did collect this type of information often did not use multivariate analysis to control for these factors in the final evaluation of impact.

Because food-based interventions are generally not amenable to experimental designs (randomized, double-blind, placebo-control trials), detailed information on potentially confounding factors is essential to ensure that the findings can indeed be attributed to the intervention. For findings to be plausible, researchers must demonstrate that an intervention had an effect above and beyond other external influences that may also have affected the outcome (Habicht, Victora, and Vaughan 1999). This is achieved by effectively controlling for potential confounding factors and biases through careful evaluation design and selection of comparison groups and appropriate multivariate data analysis methodologies. Detailed information on intermediary outcomes can also help confirm the plausibility that the final outcome is the result of the intervention. For example, an increase in serum retinol following an intervention will be more plausible if it is accompanied by a demonstrated increase in vitamin A intake.

Recommendation: Nonexperimental designs require careful collection of information on potential confounding factors and intermediary outcomes in order to demonstrate plausibility, that is, that the outcome was likely to have been caused by the intervention. Information on confounding factors and intermediary outcomes must be analyzed using appropriate multivariate analyses to control for these characteristics and to document the mechanisms by which the intervention achieved its impact.

For more information on evaluation design and analysis, see Habicht, Victora, and Vaughan 1999; Levinson et al. 1999; Rossi, Freeman, and Lipsey 1999.

Iron

Compared with vitamin A, production and education interventions to increase the supply and intake of iron from plant foods have not been popular. This is not surprising since researchers have long questioned the potential for plant sources to make a major contribution to the control of iron deficiency in developing countries (Yip 1994; De Pee et al. 1996). Although many plant foods contain relatively large amounts of iron, the nonheme form of iron in these foods has poor bioavailability. In addition, plant foods often contain a variety of compounds such as tannins, phytates, and polyphenols that inhibit the absorption of nonheme iron. Many researchers believe that it is essential to increase the household supply of more readily absorbed heme iron (found in meat and fish) by promoting the production of animal products through small animal husbandry and fish ponds. Table 1 includes a few recent experiments in this direction. In fact, of the 14 new studies reviewed, all of those that targeted increased iron intake or improved iron status encouraged the production and consumption of animal products. The study in Viet Nam, for example, promoted fish ponds and animal husbandry (English et al. 1997); the Peru intervention increased availability and awareness of low-cost sources of heme iron such as organ meats (Carrasco Sanez et al. 1998); a Bangladesh study promoted the adoption of fish ponds (IFPRI et al. 1998); and in Thailand, a home gardening intervention also supported fish ponds and chicken production along with vegetable production (Smitasiri and Dhanamitta 1999).

Impact on Iron Intake and Iron Status. The Viet Nam project documented an increase in the intake of iron among children of households in the intervention communities (home gardens, fish ponds, and animal husbandry), compared with control communities (English et al. 1997; English and Badcock 1998). No mention was made, however, of whether the increased iron was from vegetable or animal sources. Furthermore, iron status was not measured. In Peru (Carrasco Sanez et al. 1998), an effort to improve the quality of the meals offered at the community kitchens had a significant impact on the intake of foods rich in iron and vitamin C (which increases absorption of iron). The targeted group of women of reproductive age increased their total daily intake of vitamin C and heme iron and the proportion of absorbable iron consumed. The prevalence of anemia among participating women was also reduced significantly. In Bangladesh (IFPRI et al. 1998), preliminary results from a project encouraging the adoption of fish ponds or commercial vegetable production suggest that there was no increase in the intake of fish or vegetables among members of adopting households, nor was their iron status improved. This evaluation is ongoing, and longer-term impacts will be assessed.

In Thailand, preschoolers, school children, and lactating women in the intervention communities increased their iron intake as a result of a social marketing intervention. Lactating women in the intervention communities also had a greater increase in their intake of vitamin C than women in the control communities (Smitasiri and Dhanamitta 1999; Smitasiri et al. 1999). Biochemical indicators of iron status, measured only among school girls, showed significant improvements in serum ferritin. Unfortunately, the effects of the food-based intervention could not be separated from the effects of the overall strategy targeted to school girls, which included the weekly distribution of iron tablets for 12 weeks and improved the dietary quality of school lunches (Smitasiri and Dhanamitta 1999).

In Ethiopia, preliminary results of a program to commercialize the raising of crossbred cows found a 72 percent increase in household income among adopters, while their food expenditures increased by only 20 percent (Ahmed, Jabbar, and Ehui 2000). Intake of both vitamin A and iron was higher among adopters, but the authors did not differentiate between animal and plant sources of the micronutrients. Forthcoming analyses of the data will assess the impact on children's nutritional status.

Conclusions on Iron Strategies. Clearly, experience with food-based approaches to increase production and consumption of iron-rich foods is limited. Because absorption of iron from plant sources is low, efforts to reduce iron deficiency have centered on increasing the availability of heme iron. But experiences with projects to increase animal production suggest that households often face a trade-off between increased income from selling home-produced animal products and increasing their own consumption of these products. Evidence from household studies in Bangladesh (IFPRI et al. 1998) and Ethiopia (Ahmed, Jabbar, and Ehui 2000) indicates that increases in income through the sale of animal products may not significantly improve dietary quality. The results of both studies are preliminary but reinforce the observation that promoting animal production without a strong nutrition education component may not be sufficient to achieve improved dietary diversity. Households may choose to improve their income rather than their diet, and the increases in income may be invested in basic necessities other than food. Thus the question of what exactly can be achieved through well-designed integrated production and education interventions to promote increased intake of animal products and to improve iron status remains largely unanswered.

Strategies to Increase Retention of Vitamin A during Processing and Conservation

Various home-processing techniques can be used to ensure the retention of provitamin A carotenoids during food preparation, cooking, and preserving. These techniques represent another important strategy to maintain adequate vitamin A intake levels. Foods rich in provitamin A carotenoids, such as fruits and vegetables, are often highly seasonal. Home preservation techniques such as solar drying[6] and the preparation of leaf concentrates can be used to maintain a constant supply of vitamin A-rich foods and to reduce seasonal variations in availability.

Effects of Cooking and Processing on the Retention of Provitamin A

Provitamin A carotenoids are easily destroyed by exposure to light and during processing, heating, and storage, but clear estimates of the net retention rate of vitamin A with different processing techniques are not available (Rodriguez-Amaya 1997). What is known, however, is that heat treatments such as deep frying, prolonged cooking, and baking, and a combination of multiple preparation and processing methods result in substantial losses of provitamin A carotenoids. The retention of provitamin A decreases with heat treatments in the following order: microwaving is the least harmful, followed by steaming, boiling, and sautéing. Irrespective of the cooking method, retention always decreases with longer processing time, higher temperatures, and cut or macerated food. But simple modifications such as cooking with the lid on, reducing the time lag between peeling or cutting and cooking, and limiting the overall cooking, processing, and storage time can improve retention (Rodríguez-Amaya 1997).

Research is under way to resolve some of the conflicting evidence about the effects of processing on the retention of provitamin A and to standardize the methods used to analyze the vitamin A content of foods.

Appropriate Preservation Techniques Can Increase Availability throughout the Year

Vitamin A is found in large amounts in only a few foods, many of which are highly seasonal, such as oranges, noncitrus fruits and dark green, leafy vegetables. Although vitamin A is stored in the liver, the amounts ingested during the season of abundance may not be sufficient to maintain adequate vitamin A status throughout the year. Also, postharvest losses are often substantial for some vitamin A-rich foods: mangoes, for example, which ripen quickly and often all at the same time, so that the population cannot consume all the available fruit over the short period when they are available. Therefore, techniques to preserve provitamin A-rich foods must be developed and applied to ensure an adequate supply throughout the year and to reduce postharvest losses. Methods include solar drying and the production of leaf concentrates (Solomons and Bulux 1997). This latter method has the advantage of reducing the volume of the leaves and increasing the concentration of provitamin A carotenoids. This is particularly useful for young infants who have high nutrient

---

[6]The solar drying process, which is different from sun drying, will be described subsequently.

requirements and a small gastric capacity. Leaf concentrates have been used in the formulation of special complementary foods for young children and nutrient-dense flours for pregnant and lactating women.

Solar drying, one of the most popular preservation methods for fruits and vegetables rich in provitamin A, has been promoted in many countries in recent years. Solar drying is an improved alternative to the traditional sun drying method, which results in significant losses of b-carotene (provitamin A) due to direct exposure to sunlight. With solar drying, foods are dried in the shade, and high air temperatures and low humidity are provided in order to hasten the drying rate, thus retaining more provitamin A and reducing the final moisture content. This increases the micronutrient concentration in the dried products and enables the products to be stored longer. That solar-dried fruits and vegetables retain more b-carotene than sun-dried fruits and vegetables is well documented (Linehan 1994). Although the rate of retention varies for different products, the range for solar drying is 50 to 80 percent (FAO and International Life Sciences 1997). Steam blanching before solar drying has been shown to reduce overall losses during drying and storage by inactivating certain degrative enzymes (Rodriguez-Amaya 1997).

Solar drying has been promoted in a number of developing countries in recent years (IVACG 1993). In the Dominican Republic, Haiti, Mali, Senegal, and Tanzania, the feasibility of implementing solar dryers using locally available products has been demonstrated and the retention of provitamin A throughout the drying and preservation period has been assessed, mostly by VITAL (Lineham 1994). A project, carried out by the International Center for Research on Women and Opportunities for Micronutrients Interventions (OMNI), implemented and evaluated solar drying in Tanzania (Mulokozi et al. 2000). The intervention included promotion of solar dryers, nutrition and health education, and business training to facilitate the sale of dried vegetables and fruits. Solar drying was expected to increase intake of vitamin A-rich foods among preschoolers because dried foods could be available year-round; to change knowledge, attitudes, and practices through the education and behavior change components; and to increase income through the sale of surplus dried products. The study showed a slow but steady adoption rate for solar dryers (8 percent overall in intervention communities), but the percentage of households selling dried vegetables and generating income from the sale of products was small. Preschoolers' intake of vitamin A-rich foods (measured with the Helen Keller International food frequency questionnaire) increased significantly in intervention communities, compared with control communities, and differences were even larger when adopters were compared with nonadopters within intervention communities. But the increase in intake of vitamin A-rich foods mainly seems to have come from a marked increase in consumption of animal products, mainly dried sardines, as promoted by the nutrition education component, rather than from increased consumption of dried vegetables resulting from the adoption of solar dryers.

To our knowledge, the nutritional impact of similar initiatives to increase consumption of new products, such as "sweet potato buds" in Guatemala (Solomons and Bulux 1997) and leaf concentrates in Sri Lanka (Cox et al. 1993) and India (IVACG 1993) has not been evaluated.[7] As in the case of solar dryers, these technologies aim at processing foods rich in provitamin A carotenoids to concentrate and preserve their content during storage. The feasibility of these approaches at the community level and their sustainability over time, however, are being questioned (Solomons and Bulux 1997). An evaluation of a leaf concentrate production project in Sri Lanka indicated various problems with implementation of the technology at the community level, and the methodology was found to be unsustainable (Cox et al. 1993). Among other things, the machinery involved was expensive and unpopular. Women lacked motivation to use it because they found it too time consuming. More of these types of evaluations should be carried out to determine whether these apparently promising approaches can survive beyond the pilot project level, and whether they significantly contribute to reducing vitamin A deficiency.

Cooking in Iron Pots

Cooking in iron pots has long been recognized as a way to increase the iron content of food (Brittin and Nossaman 1986). Two different experimental trials tested the effectiveness of promoting the use of iron cooking pots on the iron status of young children. The first study was carried out in Brazil over a period of eight months on premature four-month-old children (Borigato and Martinez 1998). The second study was done in Ethiopia over a 12-month period on children two to five years old (Adish et al. 1999). Both studies showed statistically significant improvements in hematologic values, including iron stores. Moreover, the iron added to food cooked in iron pots was found to be bioavailable (Borigato and Martinez 1998). The laboratory analysis from the Ethiopian study found five times more iron available in meat and vegetables cooked in iron pots than in the same meal cooked in an aluminum pot. In Ethiopia, the cost of providing iron pots to a population of 10,000 (with an average family size of six) was $5,000, compared with an estimated cost ranging from $8,000 to $20,000 to provide iron supplements to women from a similar population pool for one year (Levin 1986). The authors conclude that iron pots are a relatively low-cost and sustainable way to increase the iron intake and status of deficient populations (at least of young children). They caution that the potential toxicity of using iron pots among iron-replete populations needs to be researched (Adish et al. 1999).

---

[7] Leaves that have been made into concentrates include amaranth, baobab, cassava, cowpea, sugarbeet, cauliflower, and cabbage.

Chapter 4

Strategies to Increase the Bioavailability of Micronutrients, with Emphasis on Nonheme Iron

Various home processing techniques can be used to increase the bioavailability of nonheme iron. These include fermentation or germination techniques and food-to-food fortification. Certain combinations of foods, when eaten together, promote nonheme iron bioavailability either by increasing substances that enhance absorption of iron or decreasing substances that inhibit absorption.[8] This is one form of food-to-food fortification.

Home-Processing Techniques to Reduce Inhibitors of Nonheme Iron Absorption

As indicated earlier, nonheme iron from cereals or other plants is poorly absorbed because of the presence of inhibitors of iron absorption, particularly phytic acid. Various food-processing techniques that have traditionally been used in meal preparation in Africa, Asia, and Latin America do reduce the phytic acid content of plant-based staples. Some techniques such as fermentation, germination, or malting involve enzymatic hydrolysis—a chemical breakdown—of phytic acid, whereas other nonenzymatic methods such as thermal processing, soaking, or milling can also reduce the concentration of phytic acid in some plant staples. Detailed information about these methods and their effect on improving nonheme iron bioavail-

[8]Although withholding inhibitors of iron absorption is not strictly speaking a "food-to-food fortification" approach, it is discussed here because it refers to changes in dietary patterns that can be used to improve the bioavailability of nonheme iron.

ability is available in the literature (Allen and Ahlwalia 1997; Miller 1998; Gibson and Ferguson 1998; Svanberg 1995). Only a brief summary is provided here.

Enzymatic Hydrolysis of Phytic Acid

Enzymatic hydrolysis of phytic acid in whole grain cereals and legumes can be achieved by soaking, germination, or fermentation. These processes enhance the activity of endogenous or exogenous phytase enzymes (Lorenz 1980; Chavan and Kadam 1989).

Soaking is known to increase the amount of soluble iron. For example, soaking flour for 24 hours increases the amount of soluble iron up to 10-fold (Svanberg 1995). Under optimal pH conditions, soaking wheat or rye flour for two hours completely hydrolyzes (decomposes) phytic acid (Sandberg and Svanberg 1991).

Germination consists of soaking seeds in water in the dark for up to three days to promote sprouting. During the germination process, activity of the enzyme phytase increases, causing the phytic acid to break down. Germination also reduces other antinutrients, including polyphenols and tannins. The amount of certain vitamins, including riboflavin, B_6, and vitamin C increases during germination, as well as the bioavailability of calcium, iron, and zinc (Sandberg 1991; Camacho et al. 1992). Seeds that are commonly germinated in developing countries include lentils, peas, soybeans, and mung beans.

Fermentation improves the bioavailability of minerals such as iron and zinc as a result of phytic acid hydrolysis. It also has other nutritional advantages such as increasing the content of riboflavin and vitamin B_{12} (ILSI 1998).[9] There is also some evidence that fermented foods have antidiarrheal effects in children (Mensah et al. 1990). And fermentation is a time-saver for mothers, since family members can safely eat fermented foods throughout the day. Acid or alcoholic fermentation can be used for cereals, legumes, or vegetables to increase their nutrition value and improve their physical characteristics. Fermentation can be spontaneous (using the microorganisms that are naturally present in food) or started with an inoculation.

Combining fermentation, soaking, and germination techniques is also a highly efficient way to activate endogenous phytase enzymes to degrade phytic acid and to reduce, to some extent, the amount of polyphenols that inhibit nonheme iron absorption (Svanberg 1995). Sourdough leavening and other yeast treatments, for instance, can completely degrade phytic acid.

---

[9]During fermentation, some microorganisms synthesize vitamin B_{12}, thus increasing the content available in plant-derived foods, where it is normally not present.

Nonenzymatic Methods for Reducing Phytic Acid Content

Nonenzymatic methods, such as thermal processing, soaking, and milling can also be used to reduce the phytic acid content of plant-based staples. Soaking reduces the phytic acid content of certain legumes and cereals that contain water-soluble sodium or potassium phytate (Cheryan 1980). Milling helps reduce the phytic acid content of cereals with phytic acid localized in a specific part of the grain: in maize, for example, phytic acid is found in the germ, whereas it is located in the aleurone layer of wheat, triticale, rice, sorghum, and rye (O'Dell, de Bowland, and Koirtyohann 1972). This strategy, however, also results in significant losses of vitamins and minerals (iron among others), which are also found in the aleurone layer or germ.

Experience with Home-Processing Techniques

Several studies have been carried out to develop complementary food mixtures using germination and malting techniques at home, also referred to as the amylase-rich food technology (Gopaldas et al. 1986; Mosha and Svanberg 1990; Hansen et al. 1989; Pederson et al. 1989; Singhavanich et al. 1999; Allen and Ahluwalia 1997). Using these techniques, cereal grains are sprouted, dried, and then ground into flour. Amylase—an enzyme that breaks down starch and reduces its water-holding capacity—is activated during germination. Hence only small amounts of flour are needed to reduce the viscosity of thick porridges. Interest in this technology has been driven by the need to reduce the viscosity, while maintaining the nutrient density, of complementary food mixtures for young infants who have limited gastric capacity (Gopaldas et al. 1986; Brown and Begin 1993).

A number of studies have documented reductions in viscosity and improved nutrient density of amylase-rich foods. Other studies have looked at related aspects, such as preparation time, cost, and sensory appeal (Gopaldas et al. 1986; Pederson et al. 1989; Hansen et al. 1989; Mosha and Svanberg 1990; Singhavanich et al. 1999). The impact of amylase-treated diets (or malt-treated diets) on children's dietary intake has also been summarized in a review paper (Ashworth and Draper 1992), which concludes that there was no consistent evidence of an impact on children's total energy intake. Only a few community trials have tested the acceptability of the products to mothers and children and measured the success of promotional efforts on adoption rates and sustainability over time (Vaidya 1988; Gopaldas et al. 1991; Guptil et al. 1993; Kibona et al. 1995). To our knowledge, there have been no efficacy or effectiveness studies of the impact of amylase-rich foods on the nutritional or micronutrient status of weaning-age infants, the main target group of these interventions.

Gibson et al. (1998) initiated a participatory community trial designed to combat iron, zinc, and vitamin A deficiency in Malawi, using an integrated approach that combines a variety of the strategies described earlier. The community selected the specific interventions that were to be promoted in the project. The acceptability and feasibility of the intervention was based on careful consideration of the social, cultural, economic, and environmental conditions in the communities where the project would be implemented. The set of interventions included (1) agricultural and horticultural activities to promote the production of sunflower seeds, ground nuts, soybeans, and vitamin A-rich foods, including green, leafy vegetables; (2) food preservation and processing methods such as solar drying and sunflower oil pressing to increase availability and intake of provitamin A and fat; and (3) the promotion of fermentation to enhance the content and bioavailability of micronutrients in the diet. This integrated approach was also combined with an intensive social marketing and communication strategy to promote changes in knowledge, attitudes, and practices and to achieve sustained changes in behavior. The forthcoming evaluation of this project will contribute immensely to understanding the potential of integrated food-based strategies to alleviate micronutrient malnutrition in young children and mothers.

Food-to-Food Fortification (or Dietary Combinations)

In this review, food-to-food fortification strategies to improve iron nutrition modify the diet either by including in a meal foods that promote the absorption of nonheme iron or by excluding foods that inhibit nonheme iron absorption.

Increasing the Intake of Enhancers of Nonheme Iron Absorption

In this strategy, foods containing substances that enhance nonheme iron absorption, such as fruits or vegetables rich in ascorbic acid, are eaten at the same meal as nonheme iron (Monsen 1988). Meat and fish consumed even in small amounts are also known to markedly increase nonheme iron absorption. The total iron absorbed from a typical Latin American diet based on maize and beans, for example, can be improved by the same magnitude by adding either 75 grams of meat or 50 milligrams of ascorbic acid to the diet (Svanberg 1995). Although adding small amounts of meat or fish to the diet seems like a desirable way to increase the bioavailability of nonheme iron, in reality, economic, cultural, or religious factors often hamper the effectiveness of this approach in developing countries.

One intervention promoting increased intake of meat products is the behavioral change component of the *comedores populares* program in Peru (Carrazco Sanez et al. 1998). Women were encouraged to incorporate into their diets low-cost sources of heme iron such as organ meats; this intervention proved acceptable to the women and successful in improving their iron status.

In another study, part of an ongoing Global Livestock Collaborative Research Support Program in Kenya, the impact of including small amounts of animal products in school lunches is currently being evaluated in a randomized efficacy trial (Johnson 2000). Children from 12 Kenyan elementary schools have been randomly assigned to one of four groups. For a school meal, the first group receives a serving of *githeri* (a vegetable stew of maize, beans, greens, and a small amount of fat). The second group is given *githeri* with a small amount of finely ground meat added to the stew. The third group receives 250 milliliters of milk along with a serving of *githeri*. The fourth group, a control group, receives no school meal, but families will be compensated with donated foodstuffs at the end of the trial. The effects of this animal product intervention are being evaluated for a variety of outcomes, including behavioral and cognitive abilities, anthropometry, morbidity, and biochemical indicators of micronutrient status. This carefully designed and implemented study should provide invaluable information on the impact on health, development, nutrition, and micronutrient status of school children of adding even small amounts of animal products to their diet.

The effectiveness of using ascorbic acid to improve body iron stores has been tested in a few prospective studies summarized by Svanberg (1995). These experiments, however, used vitamin C supplements, as opposed to food sources of vitamin C, and thus are not considered food-based approaches. A recent community trial carried out in rural Mexico tested the efficacy of serving fresh lemonade (as a source of ascorbic acid) with a maize, beans, and salsa meal to improve the bioavailability of iron in the diet of nonanemic, iron-deficient women (Garcia et al. in press). The study showed that 25 milligrams of ascorbic acid (in the form of lemonade) consumed at two meals a day for eight months did not significantly improve iron status. This finding was unexpected since earlier studies carried out over a 14-day period had shown a doubling of iron absorption from the addition of ascorbic acid to the typical meal. Additional efficacy trials are needed to better understand the potential and feasibility of interventions to promote greater intake of nonheme iron enhancers.

Reducing the Intake of Inhibitors of Nonheme Iron

Another dietary modification that can improve nonheme iron absorption is to reduce the intake with meals of foods and beverages that inhibit absorption of iron. For example, drinking coffee and tea one to two hours after a meal, instead of with the meal, can significantly reduce the inhibitory effect of these beverages. Consumption of only one cup of tea of normal strength has been shown to reduce iron absorption from bread or a rice with potato and onion soup by as much as 60 percent (Disler et al. 1975).

In Costa Rica, women who drank three or more cups of coffee per day during pregnancy and lactation were more likely than noncoffee drinkers to be anemic and to have infants with low iron status (low hemoglobin and hematocrit values) one month after birth (Muñoz et al. 1998). Mothers from both groups were similar in socioeconomic status, maternal anthropometry, diet, and intake of prenatal supplements. A recent study carried out in Guatemala tested the effects of reducing coffee intake on growth, morbidity, and iron status of iron-deficient toddlers (Dewey et al. 1997a, 1997b). In Guatemala, sweetened coffee with bread is a popular breakfast meal served to children, starting as early as four to six months of age. The trial randomly allocated iron-deficient toddlers into two groups: one continued to consume coffee and the other received a substitute drink containing sugar and coloring. The study documented no effects on iron status when coffee was withheld, except among children who were taking iron supplements (Dewey et al. 1997b). Among this group, serum ferritin concentrations doubled when coffee was withheld. Iron status did not change among the children who continued to drink coffee. However, a small, positive effect on growth was observed when coffee was discontinued among children who had been consuming more than 100 milliliters of coffee per day (Dewey et al. 1997a). The authors interpret the lack of significant impact of withholding coffee on iron status as being related to the relatively small amounts of coffee ingested by these children. They also speculate that the inhibitory effect of coffee on iron absorption may not be sufficient to impair iron status at all ages, and that it may be more pronounced among other more vulnerable groups, such as pregnant women.

Oregano, red sorghum, spinach, and cocoa should also be avoided with meals mainly consisting of foods of vegetable origin because they contain a substance called galloyl phenol, which is known to inhibit absorption of nonheme iron (Gibson 1997). Again, there is very little evidence available to determine whether care in combining foods and beverages in a meal is an effective way to improve iron status among poor populations in the developing world. Evidence of the efficacy of this type of intervention in a variety of age groups, populations, and individuals with different physiological statuses is urgently needed.

Some Conclusions

Two facts are strikingly clear from this review. On the one hand, technologies do exist to address some of the main concerns about the bioavailability of nonheme iron. Many of these technologies seem to involve simple, low-cost home-processing techniques, which in some cases are even part of the traditional background of the target populations. On the other hand, efforts to promote, implement, or evaluate the available technologies in community trials or in large-scale interventions have been surprisingly few. It is not clear why this is the case, but surely the scarcity of funding for program research and implementation in this area is a main constraint.

Chapter 5

Plant Breeding Strategies

Traditionally plant breeding has been used primarily to improve farm productivity, usually by developing crops with higher yields. When crossing varieties with particular traits, scientists also attempt to monitor and maintain consumer characteristics such as taste, cooking qualities, and appearance. These characteristics are important because they have a bearing on market prices, and consequently on profitability, which motivates farmers to adopt the improved varieties. Until recently, breeding to enhance the nutrient content of crops to improve human nutrition was rarely an explicit research objective, largely because it was presumed that nutrient-enhanced crops would be lower yielding, thus jeopardizing profitability and discouraging adoption by farmers. Recent research, however, indicates that at least in the case of trace minerals (iron and zinc, in particular), the objectives of breeding for higher yield and better human nutrition do largely coincide. That is, mineral-dense crops offer various agronomic advantages, such as greater resistance to infection (which reduces dependence on fungicides), greater drought resistance, and greater seedling vigor, which in turn, is associated with higher plant yield (Graham and Welch 1996). With these new developments, one of the most serious barriers to combining human nutrition and plant breeding objectives has been lifted.

The possibilities of improving micronutrient nutrition through plant breeding are numerous. They include (1) increasing the concentration of minerals (iron or zinc) or vitamins (b-carotene) in plants; (2) reducing the amount of antinutrients such as phytic acid; and (3) raising the levels of sulfur-containing amino acids, which can promote the absorption of zinc. This chapter summarizes the potential nutritional benefits of each of these approaches and updates progress in this area. More detailed information can be found in the literature (Graham and Welsh 1996; Ruel and Bouis 1998; Bouis 1996; Bouis 2000; Graham, Welch, and Bouis 2001).

Increasing the Mineral or Vitamin Concentration of Staple Crops

The main question about the potential benefits of using mineral- or vitamin-dense staple crops is whether the increased concentrations will in fact result in significant increases of bioavailable minerals (or vitamins) and consequently improve the nutritional status of deficient populations. For this to happen, vulnerable groups have to consume the improved varieties of staple crops in sufficient quantities, but even more important, the net amount of *bioavailable* nutrients they ingest must be increased relative to traditional crops.

As indicated previously, the main sources of iron in impoverished populations are staple cereals and starchy roots, tubers, and legumes. Most of the iron ingested is in the form of nonheme iron and thus has low bioavailability (Gibson 1994). Estimates indicate that cereals contribute up to 50 percent of iron intakes among households from lower socioeconomic groups (Bouis 1996). For zinc, the contribution from plant sources can be as high as 80 percent, as shown for preschoolers in Malawi (Ferguson et al. 1989). This means that doubling the iron or zinc density of food staples could increase total intakes by at least 50 percent. The main problem, though, is that diets based on plant staples usually contain large amounts of phytic acid (Gibson 1994; Allen et al. 1992), which inhibits both nonheme iron and zinc absorption. Some scientists argue that in circumstances where phytic acid is so prominent in the diet, raising the concentration of minerals in plants through plant breeding may not be sufficient to counteract the inhibitory effect of phytic acid on mineral absorption. Even if, for instance, the nonheme iron concentration of a grain is increased two- to fourfold, they argue that there may still be enough phytic acid to bind the extra minerals, in which case the net absorption of iron would not be increased.

Results based on tests on rats suggest that the percentage of bioavailability remains constant when traditional crops are compared with mineral-enhanced crops and that the final result is a net increase in bioavailable mineral. Rats, however, have substantially more intestinal phytase activity than humans (by a factor of about 30) and, therefore, rats are better able to absorb iron or zinc from high phytate foods than humans (Iqbal, Lewis, and Cooper 1994). Human bioavailability studies are urgently needed to address this critical question.

To date, most of the progress in developing mineral-dense staple crops has come from screening for genetic variability in the concentration of trace minerals. The crops tested (wheat, maize, rice, and beans) have shown significant genotypic variation, up to twice that of common cultivars for minerals (Bouis 2000; Graham, Welch, and Bouis 2001). Even greater variation has been found in the b-carotene concentration of cassava (Iglesias et al. 1997) and sweet potatoes (Hagenimana et al. 1997). The positive correlations between mineral concentrations found in grains indicate that varieties with greater iron concentration are most likely to also contain greater concentrations of zinc (Bouis 2000).

Increasing ferritin in the seed is another plant breeding approach that has the potential to increase the content of bioavailable iron in plant foods (Theil, Burton, and Beard 1997). The approach is promising because ferritin, a common source of stored iron in seeds and developing plants, appears to be highly bioavailable (Theil, Burton, and Beard 1997). New genetic engineering experiments are currently being conducted with rice to increase the concentration of iron and vitamin A in the grain. For iron this approach includes (1) increasing the iron content of the rice with a ferritin transgene; (2) reducing the phytate content of cooked rice with a transgene for a heat-stable phytase (which allows enzymatic hydrolysis of phytates during cooking); (3) overexpressing the inherent iron-enhancing, cysteine-containing rice proteins (cysteine is a promoter of nonheme iron and zinc absorption) (Layrisse et al. 1984; Lucca, Hurrell, and Potrykus 2001). Iron content in the transgenic rice increases 2-fold, phytase 130-fold, and cysteine residues 7-fold. The increase in phytase activitity is sufficient to completely degrade phytic acid in a simulated digestion experiment. In experiments generating b-carotene production in rice grain, three genes have been added—two from daffodil and one from the bacterium *Erwina uredovora* (Potrykus et al. 1999).

Although encouraging, this area of research is still at an early stage of development. Much more extensive screening, genetic engineering, and testing for safety, acceptability, and organoleptic qualities such as taste, smell, and appearance must be undertaken before the potential impact on human nutrition can be assessed.

Reducing the Phytic Acid Concentration in Plants

A complementary approach to increase the concentration of plant minerals is to act directly on the main inhibitor of absorption, phytic acid. Research in humans has shown that even small amounts of phytic acid added to meals can severely inhibit absorption of nonheme iron (Sandström and Lönnerdal 1989). Although studies do not agree on the exact point at which nonheme iron absorption is significantly improved by the removal of phytic acid, some argue that almost complete removal (down to less than 10 milligrams per meal) is necessary (Hurrell et al. 1992). Another study has shown that as little as 50 milligrams of phytic acid in a meal can cause a 78 to 92 percent reduction in nonheme iron absorption (Reddy et al. 1996).

To provide an idea of the order of magnitude of the problem, daily intakes of phytic acid among preschool-age children from populations whose staple diets are based on cereals, legumes, and starchy roots and tubers are estimated to range from 600 to 1,900 milligrams, that is 200 to 600 milligrams per meal (Gibson 1994). Among Mexican adult men and women, whose diets are based on maize (tortillas), beans, and rice, intakes of phytic acid are in the order of 4,000 to 5,000 milligrams per day (Allen et al. 1992). Cereals such as whole wheat, corn, and millet contain approximately 800 milligrams of phytic acid per 100 grams of cereal.

A key issue, then, is whether plant breeding can achieve the magnitude of reduction in phytic acid that may be necessary to obtain significant improvements in absorption of both zinc and nonheme iron. If, as suggested by Raboy (1996), phytic acid in staple foods can be reduced by a factor of two-thirds, and if dietary phytic acid comes mainly from staple foods, it is likely that this strategy would affect bioavailability of both zinc and iron and possibly also calcium, manganese, magnesium, and other trace minerals at the same time.

A small pilot study was carried out recently to measure iron absorption from low-phytate maize. The improved variety contained approximately 35 percent of the phytic acid content of regular maize, but its concentration of macronutrients and minerals was unchanged (Mendoza et al. 1998). Iron absorption was almost 50 percent greater from the low-phytate maize than from the traditional maize. These results are encouraging for populations whose diets are based on maize. Efforts to reduce the phytic acid content of staple cereals even further are under way.

Increasing the Concentration of Promoter Compounds

Another potentially complementary approach to increasing the bioavailability of minerals in staple crops is to increase the concentration of specific amino acids that promote mineral absorption. These include lysine and sulfur-containing amino acids, methionine and cysteine. At this time, there is little information about the agronomic advantages or disadvantages to increasing the concentration of these amino acids in staple foods. In terms of human nutrition, it appears that only a small increase in amino acid concentration is needed to positively affect the bioavailability of iron or zinc, and such small amounts are unlikely to affect plant functions significantly (Welch 1996). Again, this is an area that is currently being researched.

Conclusions about Plant Breeding Approaches

Involving agricultural research in the fight against micronutrient malnutrition holds great promise. Because trace minerals are important not only for human nutrition but for plant nutrition as well, plant breeding has the potential to make a significant, low-cost,[10] and sustainable contribution to reducing micronutrient deficiencies, particularly mineral deficiencies, in humans. And increasing farm productivity in developing countries is an important spin-off effect. There is increasing evidence that because iron, zinc, and provitamin A have such important synergies in absorption, transport, and function in the human body, enhancing all three nutrients simultaneously could achieve maximum impact (Graham and Rossner 1999; Garcia-Casal et al. 1998). The genetic resources needed to meet this challenge are available, and research to unveil the most promising alternatives is ongoing.

[10]Estimates of the cost of plant breeding compared with other interventions to control iron deficiency are presented in Ruel and Bouis 1998.

Chapter 6

Conclusions and Recommendations for Future Research

Can food-based strategies really reduce micronutrient malnutrition? This recurring question can be asked about both iron and vitamin A and probably about other micronutrients as well. Surprisingly, the question applies to the whole range of food-based interventions reviewed, suggesting that some of the most basic information needed to determine the usefulness of these strategies is simply not available. Questions on the efficacy and effectiveness of food-based approaches remain largely unanswered, even though some strategies, such as home gardening, have been extremely popular and have been implemented in a large number of countries for decades.

Food-based strategies to control vitamin A and iron deficiencies are at different stages of development. Experience with vitamin A programs is generally more advanced than with strategies to address iron deficiency. Tables 2 and 3 provide a summary of where current knowledge stands regarding the food-based strategies reviewed for vitamin A and iron. The research that still needs to be done to achieve progress and to improve our understanding of the potential of food-based approaches is also summarized for each micronutrient and each strategy.

Strategies to Increase Production and Intake of Micronutrient-Rich Foods

Vitamin A

Until a few years ago, the potential of plant sources to control vitamin A deficiency was based on calculations made using the conventional bioconversion factor applied

Table 2. Summary of information gaps and research needs relative to the efficacy and effectiveness of food-based approaches for reducing vitamin A deficiencies

Questions	Production and education strategies to increase supply and intake	Processing techniques to increase retention	Plant breeding strategies
Efficacy			
1. Under ideal conditions, can the intervention improve vitamin A status?	Previous calculations using conventional bioconversion factors had established amounts of vegetables and fruits needed to meet daily requirements. Recent efficacy trials challenge these estimates, showing smaller effects than expected and suggesting that b-carotene in plant is less bioavailable than previously thought.	Same questions as for production/education interventions	No information available
	Research is needed to revise bioconversion factors for foods consumed in typical diets; new efficacy trials are needed to reestablish efficacy of plant foods in improving vitamin A status of different vulnerable groups.	*Same research needs as production/education strategies*	*More plant breeding research needed* *Human bioavailability trials needed*
2. What are the ideal conditions necessary to improve vitamin A status? • How much is needed? • Of which product? • For how long? • What other factors need to be taken into account? -At the host level (such as parasites, age, nutritional and health status)? -At the food level (food matrix, food preparation, composition of the diet)?	Research is currently being done which suggests that: • Bioavailability may be different in children and mothers; • Parasites must be controlled; • Fat must be present in the diet; • Bioavailability may be greater in fruits than in dark green leafy vegetables. *Continued research is needed to determine how various host and food factors affect bioavailability of carotenoids and what are the conditions that can maximize efficacy of interventions based on plant food sources.*	Same questions as for production/education interventions *Same research needs as production/education strategies*	No information available *More plant breeding research needed* *Human bioavailability trials needed*

Effectiveness			
1. What impact do these interventions have under real life conditions?	Although evaluation designs are often weak, various production and education strategies have demonstrated an impact on a variety of outcomes, including vitamin A intake and status. *Well-designed, prospective evaluation studies are needed to look at the impact of different intervention approaches on all outcomes that may be affected. Evaluations should carefully monitor mechanisms, long-term impacts, cost, and sustainability.*	No information on effectiveness of these types of interventions to improve vitamin A status *Research needed to understand potential effectiveness of techniques such as solar drying and leaf concentrates*	No information available *More plant breeding research needed* *Human bioavailability trials needed*
2. What elements of these interventions are necessary to achieve impact?	Strong education components seem to be essential for interventions to increase production or intake, although this has not been tested formally. Many strategies use integrated approaches that seem to be successful, but this does not allow the effects of specific components to be disentangled. *Research is needed to evaluate the contribution of various components of the intervention packages to the impact and to establish best intervention packages for particular situations.*	No information available *Research needed to understand potential effectiveness of techniques such as solar drying and leaf concentrates*	No information available *More plant breeding research needed* *Human bioavailability trials needed*

Note: Research needs are in italics.

Table 3. Summary of information gaps and research needs relative to the efficacy and effectiveness of food-based approaches for reducing iron deficiencies

Strategy questions	Production and education strategies to increase supply and intake	Processing Techniques to increase retention	Plant breeding strategies
Efficacy			
1. Under *ideal* conditions, can the intervention improve iron status?	Plant foods: there are serious doubts about the potential efficacy of improving iron status through plant-based foods only. *The potential to improve iron status through plant-based strategies needs to be assessed formally. Perhaps a combination of production, education and methods to increase bioavailability would be efficacious.* Animal foods: Evidence exists from developed countries that animal food consumption improves and can adequately maintain iron status.	Evidence exists that food processing techniques can improve the bioavailability of iron. The potential impact on iron status is not known. Food-to-food fortification: There is some evidence that lime juice can improve iron status. *More research is needed on the efficacy of both these strategies to improve iron status.*	Small efficacy trial tested the impact of low-phytate maize on iron absorption. Efficacy trial looking at the impact of iron-dense rice on iron status of women is about to start in the Philippines. *More plant breeding research is needed as well as human bioavailability trials.*
2. What are the *ideal* conditions necessary to improve iron status? • How much is needed? • Of which product? • For how long? • What other factors need to be taken into account? -At the host level (such as parasites, age, nutrition, health status); -At the food level (such as food preparation, diet composition, absorption inhibitors and promoters).	Plant foods: Questions have not been formally addressed. Animal foods: It is not clear how much of different animal products are needed to improve iron status of different groups. *Efficacy trials are needed to answer these questions for both plant and animal foods and for different age and physiological status groups. For animal foods, minimal requirements to improve or maintain iron status should be established because of cost issue.*	Food processing strategies: No information available. Food-to-food fortification: One pilot study shows amount of lime juice required and duration of intervention to improve ferritin levels of women. *Research is needed on ideal doses, levels, specific aspects of these strategies.*	No information available. *More plant breeding research is needed as well as human bioavailability trials.*

Effectiveness			
1. What impact do these interventions have under real life conditions?	Plant foods: No evidence of impact on iron of any plant-based intervention without a production/education component. *Effectiveness trials of plant-based strategies should be carried out once efficacy trials have established their potential for impact.* Animal foods: Although evaluation designs are often weak, a few recent production and education strategies have demonstrated an impact on iron status *Well-designed, prospective evaluation studies are needed to look at the impact of different interventions on all outcomes that may be affected. Evaluation should also monitor mechanisms, long-term impacts, cost, and sustainability.*	Food processing: Some community trials show feasibility of implementing these interventions, but no information on impact on iron status. Food-to-food fortification: No information available. *Need effectiveness trials to determine potential of these approaches to achieve impact and to be sustainable.*	No information available. *Research in this area would be premature until efficacy is demonstrated.*
2. What elements of these interventions are necessary to achieve impact?	Animal foods: A strong education component is necessary to promote increased intake of animal products. Production alone is not sufficient to achieve greater dietary diversity, and it remains to be seen whether education can overcome economic constraints related to consumption of animal products. *Evaluation research should specifically address the issue of affordability of animal products, and the trade-offs between increased income from the production and sale of products and improved household dietary quality.*	No information available.	No information available. *Research in this area would be premature until efficacy is established.*

Note: Research needs are in italics.

to all b-carotene sources (Florentino et al. 1993), which estimated the quantity of vegetables that different family members had to eat to meet their daily requirements. Based on these calculations, it was determined that families needed to cultivate only a small plot to grow enough vegetables to meet their daily requirements (Marsh 1998). Thus, it was assumed that increasing intake of provitamin A carotenoids through home gardening would be both efficacious and feasible. A recent controversy suggesting that carotenoids have much lower bioavailability than previously assumed, however, challenges these estimates and raises fundamental questions regarding the potential efficacy of all plant-based strategies to control vitamin A deficiency.

Research to revise the bioconversion factors and to quantify the concentration of bioavailable vitamin A in different foods must be pursued. More important, research is needed to better understand the bioavailability of provitamin A in foods as they are usually prepared, processed, and consumed in the traditional diets of at-risk populations. Well-controlled epidemiological trials are required to establish what can be achieved through dietary modifications and to answer questions concerning the ideal conditions necessary to achieve maximum impact. These questions include which products should be promoted, in what amounts, and for how long. And what are the roles of various factors that affect the bioavailability of provitamin A from different sources, at the host level—such as age, health, nutritional status, and presence of parasites—and at the food level—the food matrix (the way the nutrients are present in the food), food processing, and composition of the diet? Evidence continues to accumulate about the effectiveness of well-designed and carefully implemented strategies promoting increased intake or production or both of provitamin A-rich foods using social marketing and behavior change approaches. Although evaluation designs are often weak and do not allow firm conclusions about impact (see Box on page 24), there is certainly a consistent trend indicating a positive association between these interventions and vitamin A intake and status in some cases. It may be that publication bias is playing a role, in the sense that only positive studies make it to the published literature, but there are also some examples of inconclusive results in studies that have weaker designs. Thus, in spite of the lack of information about the efficacy of food-based approaches, it seems likely that well-designed food-based approaches may play an important role in the control of vitamin A deficiency.

Iron

Information gaps exist on the potential efficacy of food-based approaches that rely on plant sources to improve iron status. Nonheme iron presents even more of a challenge than provitamin A carotenoids, because the bioavailability of nonheme iron is low and plant-based diets have high concentrations of inhibitors of absorption. The ability of animal foods to control iron-deficiency is well established, and there is no doubt that animal products in the diet can improve absorption of nonheme iron as well, thus maintaining iron status at least among the least vulnerable population groups such as adult males and women beyond their reproductive years. The exact amounts of different foods required and the frequency of intake, however, are not well documented. Efficacy trials to determine the minimum requirements for animal products to control iron deficiency among different age and physiological status groups are still needed to determine the feasibility of using these approaches in low-income, iron-deficient populations.

The main concern about promoting animal products to improve iron status is their prohibitive cost for most of the populations affected by the deficiency. Therefore, additional information on the minimum amount of animal products required to complement a plant-based diet, so that enough iron is absorbed to maintain health, would be the first step toward assessing the feasibility of such approaches. The few studies that have looked at the effectiveness of promoting animal food production have encountered the predictable problem that increased income resulting from adoption of particular production strategies may not result in improved dietary quality (IFPRI et al. 1998; Ahmed, Jabbar, and Ehui 2000). Research should explore issues related to the supply and demand of animal products that affect both farmers' incomes and consumer prices. Additionally, research should look at the income and consumption trade-offs involved in animal production and how these affect the household's dietary quality. Promoting increased intake of lower-cost sources of animal foods such as liver and entrails should be further explored, since this approach was successful with the community kitchen project in Lima, Peru (Carrasco Sanez et al. 1998). However, interventions that promote animal products may be constrained by cultural and religious factors that prohibit their inclusion in the diet of many at-risk populations.

Strategies to Increase the Bioavailability of Nonheme Iron

Various food-processing techniques and food combinations exist to increase the bioavailability of nonheme iron. However, very little information exists in the literature on the efficacy of these approaches for the control of iron deficiency. It is surprising, for instance, that of all the amylase technology studies carried out to improve the dietary quality of complementary foods, none has actually tested the impact of amylase on micronutrient status (or on growth). The same is true for the food-to-food fortification approaches. Inhibitors and promotors of nonheme iron absorption have been identified, and their effects on nonheme iron absorption are well documented in the laboratory. Yet, there are no clear guidelines on what magnitude of impact can be expected from, say, substituting another drink for tea during meals or postponing coffee consumption until two hours after the meal. Also very little has been done on the feasibility and effectiveness of promoting changes in behavior to reduce the intake of inhibitor compounds or increase the intake of promoters with the meal. Again, some of these approaches may not be successful, especially in the long term, because they often require changes in deeply entrenched cultural practices. An even more basic question is what is the minimal level of change in behavior required to achieve a level of improvement in iron bioavailability that will make a difference in iron status.

Plant Breeding Strategies

Plant breeding strategies for increased micronutrient content and bioavailability are still in an early stage, and little information is available on their ultimate value to human nutrition. The only exception is a small pilot study suggesting that low-phytate maize may increase iron absorption. Additional studies on human bioavailability are needed to understand the full potential of plant breeding strategies, but this research is a first step in that direction. It is well recognized, nevertheless, that plant breeding strategies are promising because of their immense potential to improve the dietary quality of populations relying mainly on cereal staples. In addition, if new varieties are similar to traditional varieties in terms of taste and appearance, these strategies will not require any behavior changes on the part of the consumer, which relieves one of the main challenges of most food-based approaches.

Evaluation of Food-Based Approaches

The quality of the information now available to judge the effectiveness of food-based strategies for iron and vitamin A is inadequate, and evaluation designs must be improved. Food-based approaches are complex, requiring a set of integrated activities and a wide variety of inputs and outcomes to be measured. This makes the evaluation of food-based approaches more difficult and costly than evaluations of other types of interventions. By comparison, a capsule distribution program can be evaluated by designing an intervention as a double-blinded, randomized, controlled probability trial. This type of intervention simply requires measuring a few key indicators at baseline and postintervention, in placebo and treatment groups, so that inferences of causality can be generated from the evaluation results. For food-based approaches, random allocation of treatments to participants is often not feasible (at least at the household level) and double-blind interventions are not possible; therefore evaluations must be designed to demonstrate the plausibility of the conclusions rather than to establish causality (Habicht, Victora, and Vaughan 1999). This means that the evaluation design has to include the measurement of as many potentially confounding factors as possible to help demonstrate the plausibility of the findings, that is, to prove that the results obtained can be attributed to the intervention. Multivariate analyses are also required to appropriately control for these confounding factors when assessing the significance and magnitude of impact on the outcomes of interest.

Evaluations should also include a careful analysis of the role of different intervention components on all intermediary outcomes likely to be affected and should gather information to document the mechanisms involved. They should also measure the many indirect effects of the interventions such as their contributions to the diets of other family members or in overcoming other micronutrient deficiencies.

This review does not evaluate the cost-effectiveness of alternative food-based interventions because such studies are noticeably absent from the literature. A few exceptions exist, however: studies that compare a single food-based strategy to supplementation and food fortification interventions, using aggregate data (Popkin et al. 1980; Grosse and Tilden 1988; Phillips et al. 1996). Cost-effectiveness analyses of alternative food-based interventions are sorely needed, as well as studies that contrast food-based approaches with supplementation and fortification strategies. Analyses of food-based interventions should capture spillover effects and both short- and long-term costs that influence the sustainability of alternative interventions.

A Final Word

In conclusion, this review suggests that food-based interventions have been increasingly useful and successful over the past few decades. The design and implementation of these strategies have significantly improved. This work has been largely driven by nongovernmental organizations and other local institutions and has mainly targeted vitamin A deficiency. The nutrition, agriculture, and communications research communities and donors, however, have dramatically neglected this area, and this neglect is hindering further progress. To stimulate interest and generate funds for research and program implementation, basic information on efficacy is needed. Without a fundamental demonstration of efficacy, it is difficult to motivate investment in sophisticated effectiveness and evaluation trials.

Food-based approaches should be revisited and treated with the same scientific rigor as other strategies. They are an essential component of a long-term global strategy for the fight against micronutrient malnutrition: their real potential desperately needs to be explored.

References

Adish, A. A., S. A. Esrey, T. W. Gyorkos, J. Jean-Baptiste, and A. Rojhani. 1999. Effect of consumption of food cooked in iron pots on iron status and growth of young children: A randomised trial. *Lancet* 353: 712–716.

Ahmed, M. M., M. Jabbar, and S. Ehui. 2000. Household level economic and nutritional impact of market-oriented dairy production in the Ethiopian highlands. *Food and Nutrition Bulletin* 21 (4): 460–465.

Allen, L. H., and N. Ahluwalia. 1997. Improving iron status through diet. The application of knowledge concerning dietary iron bioavailability in human populations. Opportunities for Micronutrients Interventions (OMNI). John Snow, Inc./OMNI Project, Arlington, Va. U.S.A.

Allen, L. H., J. R. Backstrand, A. Chávez, and G. H. Pelto. 1992. Functional implications of malnutrition: Final report, Mexico Project. Mexico City.

Ashworth, A., and A. Draper. 1992. The potential of traditional technologies for increasing the energy density of weaning foods. World Health Organization (WHO), Geneva.

Ayalew, W., Z. Wolde Gebriel, and H. Kassa. 1999. *Reducing vitamin A deficiency in Ethiopia: Linkages with a women-focused dairy goat farming project.* Research Report No 4. International Center for Research on Women (ICRW) /Opportunities for Micronutrients Interventions (OMNI). Washington, D.C.: ICRW.

Borigato, E. V. M., and F. E. Martínez. 1998. Iron nutritional status is improved in Brazilian preterm infants fed food cooked in iron pots. *Journal of Nutrition* (128): 855–859.

Bouis, H. 1996. Enrichment of food staples through plant breeding: a new strategy for fighting micronutrient malnutrition. *Nutrition Reviews* 54: 131–137.

———. 2000. The role of biotechnology for food consumers in developing countries. In *Agricultural biotechnology in developing countries: Towards optimizing the benefits for the poor,* ed. M. Qaim, A. Krattiger, and J. von Braun. Boston: Kluwer.

Brittin, H. C., and C. E. Nossaman. 1986. Iron content of food cooked in iron utensils. *Journal of the American Diet Association* (86): 897–901.

Brown, K. H., and F. Bégin. 1993. Malnutrition among weanlings of developing countries: Still a problem begging for solutions. *Journal of Pediatric Gastroenterology and Nutrition* 17: 132–138.

Brun, T., J. Reynaud, and S. Chevassus-Agnes. 1989. Food and nutritional impact of one home garden project in Senegal. *Ecology of Food and Nutrition* 23: 91–108.

Camacho, L., C. Sierra, R. Campos, E. Guzmán, and D. Marcus. 1992. Nutritional changes caused by germination of legumes commonly eaten in Chile. *Archivos Latinoaméricanos de Nutrición* 42: 283–290.

CARE/Nepal. 1995. A study on evaluation of home gardening program in Bajura and Mahottari Districts. Katmandu, Nepal.

Carrasco Sanez, N. C., R. M. D. deUbillas, I. S. Guillén, and S. M. Ferreira. 1998. *Increasing women's involvement in community decision-making: A means to improve iron status.* Research Report No 1. International Center for Research on Women (ICRW)/Opportunities for Micronutrients Interventions (OMNI). Washington, D.C.: ICRW.

Chakravarty, I. 2000. Food-based strategies to control vitamin A deficiency. *Food and Nutrition Bulletin* 21 (2): 135–143.

Chavan, J. K., and S. S. Kadam. 1989. Nutritional improvement of cereals by fermentation. *Critical Reviews in Food Science and Nutrition* 28 (5): 349–400.

Cheryan, M. 1990. Phytic acid interactions in food systems. *Critical Reviews in Food Science and Nutrition* 13: 297–335.

Cohen, N., M. A. Jalil, H. Rahman, M. A. Matin, J. Sprague, J. Islam, J. Davidson, E. Leemhuis de Regt, and M. Mitra. 1985. Landholding, wealth and risk of blinding malnutrition in rural Bangladeshi households. *Social Science and Medicine* 21(11): 1269–1272.

Cox, D. N., S. V. Rajasuriya, P. E. Soysa, J. Gladwin, and A. Ashworth. 1993. Problems encountered in the community-based production of leaf concentrate as a supplement for pre-school children in Sri Lanka. *International Journal of Food Sciences and Nutrition* 44: 123–132.

de Pee, S., and C. E. West. 1996. Dietary carotenoids and their role in combating vitamin A deficiency: A review of the literature. *European Journal of Clinical Nutrition* 50: S38–S53.

de Pee, S., C. E. West, Muhilal, D. Karyadi, and G. A. J. Hautvast. 1995. Lack of improvement of vitamin A status with increased consumption of dark-green leafy vegetables. *Lancet* 34: 75–81.

———. 1996. Can increased vegetable consumption improve iron status? *Food and Nutrition Bulletin* 17 (1): 34–36.

de Pee, S., M. W. Bloem, J. Gorstein, M. Sari, Satoto, R. Yip, R. Shrimpton, and Muhilal. 1998a. Reappraisal of the role of vegetables in the vitamin A status of mothers in Central Java. *American Journal of Clinical Nutrition* 68: 1068–1074.

de Pee, S., M. W. Bloem, Satoto, R. Yip, A. Sukaton, R. Tjiong, R. Shrimpton, R. Muhilal, and B. Kodyat. 1998b. Impact of a social marketing campaign promoting dark-green leafy vegetables and eggs in Central Java, Indonesia. *International Journal of Vitamin Nutrition Research* 68: 389–398.

Dewey, K. G., M. E. Romero-Abal, J. Quan de Serrano, J. Bulux, J. M. Peerson, P. Engle, and N. Solomons. 1997a. A randomized intervention study of the effects of discontinuing coffee intake on growth and morbidity of iron-deficient Guatemalan toddlers. *Journal of Nutrition* 127: 306–313.

———. 1997b. Effects of discontinuing coffee intake on iron status of iron-deficient Guatemalan toddlers: A randomized intervention study. *American Journal of Clinical Nutrition* 66: 168–176.

Disler, P. B., S. R. Lynch, R. W. Charlton, J. D. Torrance, and T. H. Bothwell. 1975. The effect of tea on iron absorption. *Gut* 16: 193–200.

English, R., and J. A. Badcock. 1998. A community nutrition project in Viet Nam: Effects on child morbidity. *Food, Nutrition and Agriculture* 22: 15–21.

English, R., J. Badcock, Tu Giay, Tu Ngu, A. M. Waters, and S. A. Bennett. 1997. Effect of nutrition improvement project on morbidity from infectious diseases in preschool children in Vietnam: Comparison with control commune. *British Medical Journal* 315 (November 1): 122–125.

Ensing, B., and S. Sangers. 1986. Home gardening in a Sri Lankan wet zone village: Can it contribute to improved nutrition? Wageningen, the Netherlands.

Fairweather-Tait, S. J. 1995. Bioavailability of iron. In *Iron interventions for child survival: Proceedings of the 17–18 May 1995 conference, London, Opportunities for Micronutrient Interventions,* ed. P. Nestel. Washington, D.C.: U.S. Agency for International Development and Child Development Institute.

FAO/WHO (Food and Agriculture Organization of the United Nations/World Health Organization). 1988. *Requirements of vitamin A, iron, folate and vitamin B12.* Food and Nutrition Series 23. Rome: FAO.

FAO (Food and Agriculture Organization of the United Nations) and International Life Sciences Institute. 1997. *Preventing micronutrient malnutrition: A guide to food-based approaches. A manual for policy makers and programme players.* Washington, D.C.: FAO.

Ferguson, E. L., R. S. Gibson, L. U. Thompson, and S. Ounpuu. 1989. Dietary calcium, phytate, and zinc intakes and the calcium, phytate, and zinc molar ratios of the diets of a selected group of East African children. *American Journal of Clinical Nutrition* 50: 1450–1456.

Florentino, R. F., M. R. A. Pedro, L. V. Candelaria, B. D. Ungson, R. U. Zarate, Jr., et al. 1993. *An evaluation of the impact of home gardening on the consumption of vitamin A and iron among preschool children.* Report No. IN-17. Vitamin A Field Support Project (VITAL), Arlington, Va., U.S.A.: International Science Technology Institute.

García, O. P., M. Díaz, J. L. Rosado, and L. H. Allen. In press. Ascorbic acid from lime juice does not improve iron status of iron deficient women in rural Mexico. *American Journal of Clinical Nutrition.*

García-Casal, M. N., M. Layrisse, L. Solano, M. A. Barón, F. Arguello, D. Llovera, J. Ramírez, I. Leets, and E. Tropper. 1998. Vitamin A and b-carotene can improve nonheme iron absorption from rice, wheat and corn by humans. *Journal of Nutrition* 128: 646–650.

Gibson, R. 1994. Zinc nutrition in developing countries. *Nutrition Research Review* 7: 151–173.

Gibson, R. S. 1997. Technological approaches to combating iron deficiency. *European Journal of Clinical Nutrition* 51 (supplement 4): S25–S27.

Gibson, R. S., and E. L. Ferguson. 1998. Food processing methods for improving the zinc content and bioavailability of home-based and commercially available complementary foods. In *Micronutrient interactions: Impact on child health and nutrition.* Washington, D.C.: International Life Sciences Institute Press.

Gibson, R. S., F. Yeudall, N. Drost, B. Mtitimuni, and T. Cullinan. 1998. Dietary interventions to prevent zinc deficiency. *American Journal of Clinical Nutrition* 68 (supplement): 484S–487S.

Gillespie, S. 1998. *Major issues in the control of iron deficiency.* Ottawa, Ont., Canada: The Micronutrient Initiative and UNICEF.

Gillespie, S., and J. Mason. 1994. Controlling vitamin A deficiency. ACC/SCN State-of-the-art series. Nutrition Policy Discussion Paper No. 14. Geneva: United

Nations Administrative Committee on Coordination—Subcommittee on Nutrition.

Gopaldas, T., P. Mehta, A. Patil, and H. Gandhi. 1986. Studies on reduction in viscosity of thick rice gruels with small quantities of an amylase-rich cereal malt. *Food and Nutrition Bulletin* 8: 42–47.

Gopaldas, T., S. Deshpande, U. Vaishnav, N. Shah, P. Mehta, S. Tuteja, S. Kanani, and K. Lalani. 1991. Transferring a simple technology for reducing the dietary bulk of weaning gruels by an amylase-rich food from laboratory to urban slum. *Food and Nutrition Bulletin* 13(4), 318–327.

Graham, R. D., and J. M. Rossner. 1999. Carotenoids in staple foods: Their potential to improve human nutrition. Paper presented at a joint International Rice Research Institute/ International Food Policy Research Institute workshop on Improving Human Nutrition through Agriculture: The Role of International Agricultural Research, Los Baños, Philippines, October 5–7, 1999.

Graham, R. D., and R. M. Welch. 1996. *Breeding for staple food crops with high micronutrient density.* Working Papers on Agricultural Strategies for Micronutrients No. 3. Washington, D.C.: International Food Policy Research Institute.

Graham, R. D., R. M. Welch, and H. E. Bouis. 2001. Addressing micronutrient malnutrition through enhancing the nutritional quality of staple foods: Principles, perspectives, and knowledge gaps. *Advances in Agronomy* 70: 77–142.

Greiner, T., and S. N. Mitra. 1995. Evaluation of the impact of a food-based approach to solving vitamin A deficiency in Bangladesh. *Food and Nutrition Bulletin* 16 (3): 193–205.

Grosse, R., and R. Tilden. 1988. Vitamin A cost-effectiveness model. *International Journal of Health Planning and Management* 3: 225–244.

Guptil, K. S., S. A. Esrey, G. A. Oni, and K. H. Brown. 1993. Evaluation of a face-to-face weaning food intervention in Kwara State, Nigeria: Knowledge, trial, and adoption of a home prepared weaning food. *Social Sciences and Medicine* 36: 665.

Habicht, J.-P., C. G. Victora, and J. P. Vaughan. 1999. Evaluation designs for adequacy, plausibility and probability of public health programme performance and impact. *International Journal of Epidemology* 28: 10–18.

Hagenimana, V., M. Anyango Oyunga, J. Low, S. M. Njoroge, S. T. Gichuki, and J. Kabira. 1999. *Testing the effects of women farmers' adoption and production of orange-fleshed sweet potatoes on dietary vitamin A intake in Kenya.* Research Report No. 3. International Center for Research on Women (ICRW) /Opportunities for Micronutrients Interventions (OMNI). Washington, D.C.: ICRW.

Hallberg, L. 1981. Bioavailability of dietary iron in man. *Annual Review of Nutrition* 1: 123–147.

Hansen, M., B. Pedersen, L. Munck, and B. O. Eggum. 1989. Weaning foods with improved energy and nutrient density prepared from germinated cereals. 1. Preparation and dietary bulk of gruels based on barley. *Food and Nutrition Bulletin* 11 (2): 40–45.

HKI/AVRDC (Helen Keller International/Asian Vegetable Research and Development Institute). 1993. Home gardening in Bangladesh: Evaluation report. New York.

Howsen, C. P., E. T. Kennedy, and A. Horwitz, eds. 1998. *Prevention of micronutrient deficiencies: Tools for policymakers and public health workers.* Washington, D.C.: National Academy Press.

Hurrell, R. G., M.-A. Juillerat, M. B. Reddy, S. R. Lynch, S. A. Dassenko, and J. D. Cook. 1981. Soy protein, phytate, and iron absorption in humans. *American Journal of Clinical Nutrition* 56: 573–578.

IFPRI (International Food Policy Research Institute), Bangladesh Institute of Development Studies, Institute of Nutrition and Food Science, Data Analysis and Technical Assistance and Research Department of Human Nutrition, Royal Veterinary and Agricultural University. 1998. Commercial vegetable and polyculture fish production in Bangladesh: Their impacts on income, household resource allocation, and nutrition, vol.1. IFPRI, Washington, D.C.

Iglesias, C., J. Mayer, L. Chavez, and F. Calle. 1997. Genetic potential and stability of carotine content in cassava roots. *Euphytica* 94: 367–373.

ILSI (International Life Sciences Institute). 1998. *Micronutrient interactions: Impact on child health and nutrition.* Report of a meeting held in Washington, D.C., July 29–30, 1996. Washington, D.C.: ILSI Press.

Immink, M., D. Sanjur, and M. Colon. 1981. Home gardens and the energy and nutrient intakes of women and preschoolers in rural Puerto Rico. *Ecology of Food and Nutrition* 11: 191–199.

Institute of Medicine. 2001. Dietary reference intakes for vitamin A, vitamin K, arsenic, boron, chromium, copper, iodine, iron, manganese, molybdenum, nickel, silicon, vanadium, and zinc. Panel on Micronutrients, Subcommittees on Upper Reference Levels of Nutrients and of Interpretation and Use of Dietary Reference Intakes, and the Standing Committee on the Scientific Evaluation of Dietary Reference Intakes, Food and Nutrition Board, National Academy of Sciences, Washington, D.C.

Iqbal, T. H., K. O. Lewis, B. T. Cooper. 1994. Phytase activity in the human and rats small intestine. *Gut* 35: 1233–1236.

IVACG (International Vitamin A Consultative Group). 1993. *Toward comprehensive programs to reduce vitamin A deficiency.* Report of the 15th International Vitamin A Consultative Group Meeting, Arusha, Tanzania, March 8–12, 1993. Washington, D.C.: IVACG.

———. 1999. *Vitamin A and other micronutrients: Biologic interactions and integrated interventions.* Report of the 19th International Vitamin A Consultative Group Meeting, Durban, South Africa, March 8–11, 1999. Washington, D.C.: IVACG.

Jalal, F., M. C. Nesheim, Z. Agus, D. Sanjur, and J. P. Habicht. 1998. Serum retinal concentrations in children are affected by food sources of b-carotene, fat intake, and antihelmintic drug treatment. *American Journal of Clinical Nutrition* 68: 623–629.

Johnson, S. 2000. The role of animal source foods in improving micronutrient nutrition in Kenyan children. *SCN News* 20: 39–40.

Kibona, N., C. Doland, F. E. Watson, D. Alnwick, and A. Tomkins. 1995. An evaluation of a project to improve child nutrition in Tanzania. *International Journal of Food Sciences and Nutrition* 46: 233–239.

Kidala, D., T. Greiner, and M. Gebre-Medhin. 2000. Five-year follow-up of a food-based vitamin A intervention in Tanzania. *Public Health and Nutrition* 3 (4): 425–431.

Kuhnlein, H. V. 1992. Change in the use of traditional foods by the Nuxalk native people of British Columbia. *Ecology of Food and Nutrition* 27: 259–282.

Kuhnlein, H. V., and S. Burgess. 1997. Improved retinol, carotene, ferritin, and folate status in Nuxalk teenagers and adults after a health promotion programme. *Food and Nutrition Bulletin* 18 (2): 202–210.

Layrisse, M., C. Martinez-Torres, I. Leets, P. Taylor, and J. Ramirez. 1984. Effects of histidine, cysteine, glutathione, or beef on iron absorption in humans. *The Journal of Nutrition* 114: 217–223.

Levin, H. M. 1986. A benefit-cost analysis of nutritional programs for anemia reduction. *World Bank Research Observer* 1: 219–237.

Levinson, F. J., B. L. Rogers, K. M. Hicks, T. Schaetzel, L. Troy, and C. Young. 1999. *Monitoring and evaluation: A guidebook for nutrition project managers in developing countries.* Tools to Measure Performance of Nutrition Programs 8. Washington, D.C.: Human Development Network, the World Bank.

Linehan, M. 1994. *Assessment of food preservation activities for vitamin A nutrition.* Vitamin A Field Support Program (VITAL) Report No. IN-30. Arlington, Va., U.S.A.: International Life Science and Technology Institute.

Lorenz, K. 1980. Cereal sprouts: Composition, nutritive value, food applications. *Critical Reviews in Food Science and Nutrition* 13: 353–385.

Lucca, P., R. Hurrell, and I. Potrykus. 2001. Genetic engineering approaches to improve the bioavailability and the level of iron in rice grain. *Theoretical and Applied Genetics* 102: 392–397.

Marsh, R. 1998. Building on traditional gardening to improve household food security. *Food, Nutrition and Agriculture* 22: 4–14.

McLaren, D. S., and M. Frigg. 1997. Sight and life manual on vitamin A deficiency disorders (VADD). Task Force on Sight and Life, Basel, Switzerland.

Mendoza, C., F. E. Viteri, B. Lönnerdal, K. A. Young, V. Raboy, and K. H. Brown. 1998. Effect of genetically modified, low-phytic-acid maize on absorption of iron from tortillas. *American Journal of Clinical Nutrition* 68: 1123–1127.

Mensah, P. P., A. M. Tomkins, B. S. Drasar, and T. J. Harrison. 1990. Fermentation of cereals for reduction of bacterial contamination of weaning foods in Ghana. *Lancet* 336: 140–143.

Miller, D. D. 1998. Effects of cooking and food processing on the content of bioavailable iron in foods. In *Micronutrient interactions: Impact on child health and nutrition.* Washington, D.C.: International Life Sciences Institute Press.

Monsen, E. R. 1988. Iron nutrition and absorption: Dietary factors which impact iron bioavailability. *Journal of the American Dietetic Association* 88: 786–790.

Mosha, A. C., and U. Svanberg. 1990. Preparation of weaning foods with high nutrient density using flour of germinated cereals. *Food and Nutrition Bulletin* 5(2): 10–14.

Mulokozi, G., L. Mselle, C. Mgoba, J. K. L. Mugyabuso, and G. D. Ndossi. 2000. *Improved solar drying of vitamin A-rich foods by women's groups in the Singida District of Tanzania.* Research Program No. 5. International Center for Research on Women/ Opportunities for Micronutrient Interventions (OMNI). Washington, D.C.: ICRW.

Muñoz, L. M., B. Lönnerdal, C. L. Keen, and K. G. Dewey. 1988. Coffee consumption as a factor in iron deficiency anemia among pregnant women and their infants in Costa Rica. *American Journal of Clinical Nutrition* 48: 645–666.

O'Dell, B. L. O., A. R. de Bowland, S. R. Koirtyohann. 1972. Distribution of phytate and nutritionally important elements among the morphological components of cereal grains. *Journal of Agriculture and Food Chemistry* 20: 718.

Parlato, M., and P. Gottert. 1996. Promoting vitamin A in rural Niger: Strategies for adverse conditions. In *Strategies for promoting vitamin A production, consumption, and supplementation. Four case studies,* ed. R. E. Seidel. Washington, D.C.: Academy for Educational Development.

Pedersen, B., M. Hansen, L. Munck, and B. O. Eggum. 1989. Weaning foods with improved energy and nutrient density prepared from germinated cereals. 2. Nutritional evaluation of gruels based on barley. *Food and Nutrition Bulletin* 11(2): 46–52.

Peduzzi, C. 1990. *Home and community gardens assessment program implementation experience: The tip of the iceberg.* Vitamin A Field Support Project (VITAL) Report No. TA-2. Washington, D.C.: International Life Sciences Institute.

Phillips, M., T. Sanghvi, R. Suarez, J. McKigney, and J. Fiedler. 1996. The costs and effectiveness of three vitamin A interventions in Guatemala. *Social Sciences and Medicine* 42(12): 1661–1668.

Pollard, R. 1989. The West Sumatra vitamin A social marketing project. Department of Health, Indonesia, and Helen Keller International, New York.

Popkin, B. M., F. S. Solon, T. Fernandez, and M. C. Latham. 1980. Benefit-cost analysis in the nutrition area: A project in the Philippines. *Social Science and Medicine* 14C: 207–216.

Potrykus, I., P. Lucca, X. Ye, S. Al-Babili, R. F. Hurrel, and P. Beyer. 1999. Contributions to food security by genetic engineering with rice. Press release, August 3, 1999, St. Louis, Mo., U.S.A.

Raboy, V. 1996. Cereal low phytic mutants: A global approach to improving mineral nutritional quality. *Micronutrients and Agriculture* 2: 15–16.

Reddy, M. B., R. F. Hurrell, M. A. Juillerat, and J. D. Cook. 1996. The influence of different protein sources on phytate inhibition of nonheme-iron absorption in humans. *American Journal of Clinical Nutrition* 63: 203.

Rodríguez-Amaya, D. B. 1997. *Carotenoids and food preparation: The retention of provitamin A carotenoids in prepared, processed, and stored foods.* Opportunities for Micronutrients Interventions (OMNI) Project. Arlington, Va., U.S.A.: John Snow, Inc.

Rossi, P. H., H. E. Freeman, and M. W. Lipsey. 1999. *Evaluation: A systematic approach,* 6th ed. Thousand Oaks, Calif., U.S.A.: Sage Publications.

Ruel, M. I. T., and H. E. Bouis. 1998. Plant breeding: A long-term strategy for the control of zinc deficiency in vulnerable populations. *American Journal of Clinical Nutrition* 68(2-S): 488S–494S.

Sandberg, A. S. 1991. The effect of food processing on phytate hydrolysis and availability of iron and zinc. *Advances in Experimental Medicine and Biology* 289: 499–508.

Sandberg, A. S., and U. Svanberg. 1991. Phytate hydrolysis in cereals: Effects on in vitro estimation of iron availability. *Journal of Food Science* 56: 1330–1333.

Sandström, B., and B. Lönnerdal. 1989. Promoters and antagonists of zinc absorption. In *Zinc in human biology*, ed. C. F. Mills. Human Nutrition Reviews, International Life Sciences Institute. London: Springer-Verlag.

Singhavanich, C., S. Jittinandana, W. Kriengsinyos, and S. Dhanamitta. 1999. Improvement of dietary density by the use of germinated cereals and legumes. *Food and Nutrition Bulletin* 20 (2): 261–266.

Smitasiri, S., and S. Dhanamitta. 1999. *Sustaining behavior change to enhance micronutrient status: Community and women-based interventions in Thailand.* Research Report No. 2, International Center for Research on Women (ICRW)/ Opportunities for Micronutrients Interventions (OMNI). Washington, D.C.: ICRW.

Smitasiri, S., G. A. Attg, A.Valyasevi, S. Dhanamitta, and K.Tontisirin. 1993. Social marketing vitamin A rich foods in Thailand: A model nutrition communication for behavior change process. The Institute of Nutrition, Mahidol University, Bangkok, Thailand.

Smitasiri, S., K. Sa-ngobwarchar, P. Kongpunya, C. Subsuwan, O. Banjong, C. Chitchumroonechokchai, W. Rusami-Sopaporn, S.Veeravong, and S. Dhanamitta. 1999. Sustaining behavioural change to enhance micronutrient status through community and women-based interventions in northeast Thailand: Vitamin A. *Food and Nutrition Bulletin* 20 (2): 243–251.

Soleri, D., D. A. Cleveland, and T. R. Frankenberger. 1991. *Gardens and vitamin A: A review of recent literature.* Vitamin A Field Support Project (VITAL) Report No. IN-2. Arlington, Va., U.S.A.: VITAL, International Science Technology Institute.

Soleri, D., D. A. Cleveland, and A.Wood. 1991. *Vitamin A nutrition and gardens bibliography.* Vitamin A Field Support Project (VITAL) Report No. IN-1. Arlington, Va., U.S.A.: VITAL, International Science Technology Institute.

Solomons, N. W., and J. Bulux. 1997. Identification and production of local carotene-rich foods to combat vitamin A malnutrition. *European Journal of Clinical Nutrition* 51 (suppl. 4): S39–S45.

Solon, F., T. L. Fernández, M. C. Latham, and B. M. Popkin. 1979. An evaluation of strategies to control vitamin A deficiency in the Philippines. *American Journal of Clinical Nutrition* 32: 1445–1453.

Sommer, A., and K. P. West. 1996. *Vitamin A deficiency: Health, survival, and vision.* New York and Oxford: Oxford University Press.

Svanberg, U. 1995. Dietary interventions to prevent iron deficiency in preschool children. In *Iron interventions for child survival: Proceedings of the 17–18 May 1995 conference, London, Opportunities for Micronutrient Interventions,* ed. P. Nestel. Washington, D.C.: U.S. Agency for International Development and Institute for Child Health.

Theil, E. C., J. W. Burton, and J. L. Beard. 1997. A sustainable solution for dietary iron deficiency through plant biotechnology and breeding to increase seed ferritin control. *European Journal of Clinical Nutrition* 51: S28–S31.

UN ACC/SCN (United Nations Administrative Committee on Coordination/ Subcommittee on Nutrition). 1997. *Third report on the world nutrition situation.* Geneva: ACC/SCN.

Underwood, B. A. 2000. Dietary approaches to the control of vitamin A deficiency: An introduction and overview. *Food and Nutrition Bulletin* 21 (2): 117–123.

Vaidya, Y. 1988. Weaning foods in Nepal. In *Improving young child feeding in Eastern and Southern Africa,* ed. D. Alnwick, S. Moses, and O. G. Schmidt. Ottawa, Canada: International Development Research Center.

Welch, R. M. 1996. The optimal breeding strategy is to increase the density of promoter compounds and micronutrient minerals in seeds: Caution should be used in reducing anti-nutrients in staple food crops. *Micronutrients and Agriculture* 1: 20–22.

WHO (World Health Organization). 1995. *Global prevalence of vitamin A deficiency.* Micronutrient Deficiency Information System Working Paper 2. Geneva: WHO.

Yip, R. 1994. Iron deficiency: Contemporary scientific issues and international programmatic approaches. *Journal of Nutrition* 125: 1479S–1490S.

About the author

Marie T. Ruel is a research fellow in the Food Consumption and Nutrition Division of the International Food Policy Research Institute. She leads a multicountry research program to analyze the food security and nutrition implications of rapid urbanization in developing countries. She also conducts research on strategies to alleviate micronutrient deficiencies and methodologies to measure, quantify, and analyze the importance of maternal caregiving practices for child nutrition. Ruel received a PhD in international nutrition from Cornell University.

Made in the USA
Monee, IL
04 November 2026

67379788R00046